PRAISE FOR DR. H

I had always been reluctant to smile because of the space between my two front teeth. One picture taken at my youngest son's wedding showed my teeth and I realized just how bad they looked. My oldest son commented that I would "be so pretty" if I had the space between my teeth closed, and suggested I consult with a cosmetic dentist. I took his suggestion and scheduled a consultation with [Dr. Flax].

My first visit with [Dr. Flax] revealed that I was actually missing a tooth on both sides of [my] front teeth. In addition, there was excess tissue between these teeth, which was connected to my upper gum. While I have always had regular dental care, I had never been told this before. It was then that I decided to begin the process of correction. Now, I enjoy smiling because of my beautiful teeth.

Thanks to [Dr. Flax] and [his] wonderful staff. The care, concern, and love I received on each visit were special. In return, I want [Dr. Flax] to know how appreciative I am. I have a new "dental family," and I love each of you.

—Hazel M. Roberts
  patient

A wonderful read! Hugh is someone who understands real people, smiles, and ethics. This book is a fitting addition to his outstanding contribution to global dentistry.

—Tif Querishi, BDS

  clinical director, IAS Academy
  editorial board, Dental Update
  former president, BACD

The Moses of Dentistry, Dr. Hugh Flax! More than ten years ago, Dr. Flax changed my life.

I came to him seeking a new smile look. I wanted to eliminate a big front gap, an overbite, uneven teeth on the bottom and the top, and the dingy color. Dr. Flax met with me and showed me a picture of the expected outcome. He answered all of my questions and we agreed on the plan. Several months later, following Invisalign and impressions, Dr. Flax put the four temporary veneers on and I was so impressed! Dr. Flax gave me his cell phone number to call if I had any problems. I left the office feeling that a true miracle had been performed. My next step was to return in a week or two to get my permanent smile. I was truly a happy camper!

Several days later, on a Sunday afternoon, I broke one of the temporary veneers. I was dining with several friends when it happened. I shouted, "Oh my God, I just broke my tooth." I then said, "Let me call my dentist." One of my friends bet me $50 that my dentist would not answer the telephone on a Sunday. I took the bet! I called Dr. Flax, and he answered on the second ring and told me to meet him at the office. I got my $50 and left to meet Dr. Flax at his office. Dr. Flax fixed my temporary veneer at no charge. I later shared with him the story about the bet, and we laughed together! I returned later to Dr. Flax's office to receive my permanent smile. He did an awesome job! That's when I deemed him to be the "Moses of Dentistry!"

Everywhere I go, people talk about my beautiful smile. A day never passes without me receiving commendations on my majestic smile! Now, fast forward to March 9, 2019. I have a bad fall that resulted in several bruises and two broken teeth. I immediately sent Dr. Flax an instant message and a picture of my face. Dr. Flax responded within five minutes. Once again, Dr. flax was there for me. When my mother saw my temporary veneers, she said, "Yes, he really is the Moses of Dentistry!" I am wearing my temporary veneers and will return soon to get my new permanent smile once again. Dr. Flax is the greatest! He gives me his very best every time!

Thanks, Dr. Flax, you will always be my MOSES OF DENTISTRY!

—Dr. Frances E. Davis

chief human resources officer, Gwinnett County Public Schools
patient

Hugh is an amazing dentist with an incredible eye for details and an insatiable pursuit of learning and improving. His commitment to dentistry, his patients, and the American Academy of Cosmetic Dentistry is virtually unparalleled.

—Sandy Roth

owner, ProSynergy Dental Communications

Dr. Flax has created the guidebook to cosmetic dentistry. Tons of great information to help the cosmetic dentistry consumer ask the right questions and make the right choices. He has taken a career worth of knowledge and distilled it in a way for the general public to become a more informed patient. A great resource for anyone looking to enhance their smile!

—Gary Radz, DDS

author, lecturer on cosmetic dentistry
Denver, CO

In a day where consumers are taking an active role in their own healthcare, both information and misinformation are readily available. Dr. Hugh Flax's publication both educates consumers about the importance of quality dental care and provides valuable, sound information to help consumers make informed decisions to identify the care they deserve. Dr. Flax's willingness to share personal and professional insight gained over the life of his career is a true gift to his readers.

—W. Johnston Rowe, Jr., DDS, AAACD

former AACD accreditation chair

I first moved to Atlanta almost thirty years ago. I needed a dentist and was recommended by several coworkers to see Dr. Flax. I became one of Doc's first patients when he opened his first office. Because he was a perfectionist, I knew that I had found the right dentist for me. I have watched him continue to learn new techniques and to study new aspects of dentistry and become a leader in his field. He and his fabulous staff have given me back my perfect, healthy, beautiful, and bright smile by putting veneers over the lines and hairline cracks that were left on my teeth by wearing braces for so many years when I was younger. He must have been born compassionate, caring, and gentle, as he has saved my smile through some harrowing dental emergencies and gave me confidence that "everything will be okay" when he finished the various procedures. So proud of [him] and the fine reputation that [he has] built.

—Jan McGeough

patient
Atlanta, GA

I have had the pleasure to work with Dr. Flax for nineteen years helping to give his patients the smile of their dreams with an unmatched patient experience. What I like about Dr. Flax is his dental hand skills, attention to detail, and quest for dental education and knowledge. Our relationship has been one of collaboration and fun throughout the years. Thank you Dr. Flax for your friendship and support.

—Wayne Payne, CDT, AAACD

Payne Dental Lab
San Clemente, CA

As a dedicated practitioner on a never-ending quest for deeper knowledge, Dr. Flax brings a rare, comprehensive perspective to his clinical teachings.

—Jeffrey W. Horowitz, DMD, FAGD, DASBA

mentor, Kois Center
Conway, SC

Dr. Hugh Flax is an extremely talented cosmetic dentist and is committed to giving 110 percent to his patients and his profession.

—Todd Snyder, DDS, FAACD, FIADFE

cosmetic dentist, author, public speaker, entrepreneur
Laguna Niguel, CA

I was in need of a complete set of upper teeth due to past poor dentistry and, yes, poor dental hygiene on my part as a result of very bad experiences as a child creating a real fear of dentists. As a result, I did a lot of research to pick where I would go for my "teeth in a day."

I chose Flax Dental after much research and reading the on line reviews. I did not know anyone who had been to Flax Dental so I did not have any firsthand accounts. My first time there I was very nervous and really out right scared. Dr. Flax and his staff did their best to put me at ease and by the end of the visit, I felt assured enough to make another appointment and to keep it. From me, that is high praise indeed since previously I only went to the dentist when I was in so much pain, I didn't have a choice.

I highly recommend Dr. Flax and his whole team, including Dr. Brady and his team and Robin Johnson and his team. If you have a fear of dentists that have kept you from taking care of your teeth, I recommend Dr. Flax and team even if you don't need "teeth in a day." My guess is your experience will be like mine and you could lose, or at the very least, lessen your fear of dentists. It has taken me a lifetime to find someone that I feel like I can see on a regular basis to keep my dental heath in good shape, now restored through a team effort of myself and Flax Dental.

—**E. Pizzati**

patient

Before coming to see Dr. Flax, I had been dealing with chronic dental discomfort for around three years. During that time, I had two root canals, multiple gum treatments, and wore night guards to try to relieve the pain, but it never went away. Dr. Flax recommended I wear a deprogrammer at night for a few weeks and see if things improved, and they did. After that, he spent about an hour fixing the bite throughout my entire mouth, not just one area. I felt an improvement that day! A week later, I now have no dental pain and my periodontist noticed that my gums have improved as well—my six pocket is now a four. My only regret is not seeing Dr. Flax sooner to have this procedure done. It could have saved me years of discomfort, thousands of dollars, and unnecessary sadness and stress. When I close my mouth now, my jaw and teeth have a "happy cloud" to rest on instead of banging and knocking around. I can now spend each day focused on enjoying the day instead of worrying and wondering about my dental pain and how to make it go away. My quality of life is so much better and I love to smile now, thanks to Dr. Flax.

—Dr. Natalie Goldberger
> patient

I have worked with Dr. Flax over the past eight years and have a great admiration for his attention to detail on each case he presents. As a dental technician, I value his support of the team approach and relationship between dentist, surgeon, and technician. He exudes a wealth of knowledge and experience in various areas of the industry, and is always ready to learn more and share said knowledge. One of the best to work with!

—Robin Johnson
> RJ Dental Creations
> specializing in Teeth in a Day design

a *Smile* is Always in Style

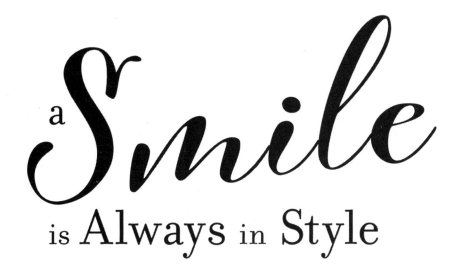

a Smile is Always in Style

HOW TO LOOK GREAT AND FEEL AMAZING

HUGH FLAX DDS, AAACD, MICOI

Advantage.

Published by Advantage, Charleston, South Carolina.
Member of Advantage Media Group.

ADVANTAGE is a registered trademark, and the Advantage colophon is a trademark of Advantage Media Group, Inc.

Printed in the United States of America.

10 9 8 7 6 5 4 3 2 1

ISBN: 978-1-64225-101-2
LCCN: 2019939620

Cover and layout design by Wesley Strickland.

This publication is designed to provide accurate and authoritative information in regard to the subject matter covered. It is sold with the understanding that the publisher is not engaged in rendering legal, accounting, or other professional services. If legal advice or other expert assistance is required, the services of a competent professional person should be sought.

Advantage Media Group is proud to be a part of the Tree Neutral® program. Tree Neutral offsets the number of trees consumed in the production and printing of this book by taking proactive steps such as planting trees in direct proportion to the number of trees used to print books. To learn more about Tree Neutral, please visit **www.treeneutral.com**.

Advantage Media Group is a publisher of business, self-improvement, and professional development books and online learning. We help entrepreneurs, business leaders, and professionals share their Stories, Passion, and Knowledge to help others Learn & Grow. Do you have a manuscript or book idea that you would like us to consider for publishing? Please visit **advantagefamily.com** or call **1.866.775.1696**.

TABLE OF CONTENTS

Your Guide to a Fearless Smile

The Importance of a Great Smile

Whitening: Truth or Consequences

Straightening—Looks Great and Preserves Your Teeth

Bonding and Contouring— A Simple Solution

Veneers Can Help You Look and Feel Younger

ACKNOWLEDGMENTS

Blessed and grateful to so many in my life who have supported my journey toward excellence and compassion:

To my dad, who was my hero and role model on so many levels.

To my family and friends, who give me strength, wisdom, and love.

To my Flax Dental team, who follow my passion.

To my many loyal patients, who have entrusted me with their smiles and longevity.

To my mentors around the world, who feed my curiosity of constant improvement.

To my spirit, that guides me on a path of kindness and integrity.

And to my beloved mom, who inspired me to become a dentist who makes a profound difference.

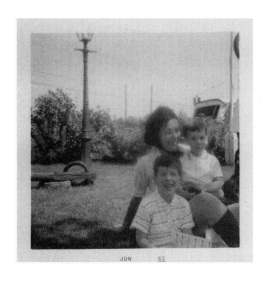

FOREWORD

She covered her mouth with her hand to make sure no one saw her laughing.

I'd watched her do it a thousand times. The first time, it seemed odd. But over the years, after I realized, she did it every time she laughed, I assumed it was because she'd been told: proper ladies don't throw their heads back with laughter. It made me sad because I believed she was afraid to express joy.

I couldn't have been more wrong.

Years later, looking at an old photograph, I saw the truth. Covering her mouth when she laughed wasn't because she was afraid of joy. It was because of her teeth.

The woman I'm describing was my mother-in-law. For the entire time I knew her, she covered her mouth when she laughed. I never understood why. Her teeth always seemed fine to me. In fact, they were quite straight. But after she died, I found some old photos of her in college. There she was standing beneath the University of Georgia arches in a beautiful white wool coat, flashing a big happy smile; she looked fabulous. Yet closer inspection of the small picture revealed that her teeth were misaligned. I asked my husband about it. He said, "My mother always had problems with her teeth. They were so bad she wound up getting dentures when she was in her fifties."

That's when the full weight of it hit me. The woman I knew, or the woman I thought I had known, the woman I assumed was afraid to express joy, had spent the first fifty years of her life embarrassed about her teeth. By the time she got dentures, the habit was so ingrained it had become part of her. She spent decades afraid to smile for photos or laugh out loud with her children. Even her wedding pictures showed a tight-lipped grin.

Her experience is not unique.

It's shocking that something as seemingly simple as your teeth can have such a dramatic impact on your life. In the course of our day-to-day lives, most of us don't think about how our teeth affect our relationships. Yet, as I saw with my mother-in-law, your smile is the way you connect. I have to wonder, over time, did her reluctance to smile affect her personality? I think it did.

Your smile is the way you convey joy, love, and acceptance. It communicates volumes to the people around you. When you don't feel confident about your smile, it affects everything about you. It affects the way you feel in any setting, and the way people respond to you.

As humans, we make snap judgments about each other based on appearances. We do it thousands of times a day. In his breakthrough book, *Blink: The Power of Thinking Without Thinking*, Malcolm Gladwell revealed that our default wiring is to think without thinking. We size up situations and determine how we feel about someone based on nothing more than two-second observations.

Much of the time, our instincts are right. But sometimes, we're dead wrong. When a person doesn't smile, we make all kinds of negative assumptions. Very rarely do we question, *I wonder if it's their teeth?*

When Dr. Flax told me he was writing a book, I was delighted. I've known Hugh Flax for almost a decade. During that time I've watched him transform the smiles of thousands of people, including my own. His office walls are lined with pictures of beaming, smiling people who are now able to go out into the world confident and happy because their smile reflects the person they are inside.

I'm honored to write the foreword for this book, because I've seen firsthand just how much your teeth matter. Your teeth affect your personal relationships, and your professional success.

As a business coach, I work with CEOs, and I can tell you almost every single one of them has a great smile. To be clear, there's not a panel of judges who says we can't promote this person because they don't smile. You won't find a requirement for straight white teeth on a corporate job description (unless you're a tooth model). And no one ever got dinged on a performance review for crooked teeth.

Yet, people are evaluated every day. We assess people on their confidence, their ability to connect with others, and how comfortable we feel in their presence. All those things start with your smile.

I wish I could go back in time and help my mother-in-law reclaim her smile. I wish she had experienced the joy and confidence that comes from a healthy smile. And more than anything, I wish she had more unfiltered, no hands required, head back, full-throated laughs with the people she cared about.

But we can't go backward. All we can do is move forward.

When Dr. Flax says, "A smile is always in style," he's right. We all deserve a great smile. This book will help you find yours.

Lisa Earle McLeod
Author, *Selling with Noble Purpose*
Founder, McLeod & More, Inc.

YOUR GUIDE TO A FEARLESS SMILE

My mom was scared about going to the dentist. If you imagine a tree in a hurricane, that's how much she shook. Oftentimes, she was given barbiturates to cope with her fears.

To make matters worse, my dad traveled for his job in the 1970s. Since Mom was always being sedated for her dental procedures, she had to drive herself to and from her appointments. Fortunately, the dentist's office was less than two miles away—and driving laws were less restrictive than they are today.

The good news was that she had a dentist who was a gentleman—and a gentle man. He rebuilt her mouth in about twelve months. I was a junior in high school at the time, and it was the first time in her life that she was able to smile and eat with confidence. I was so happy for her.

Seeing what my mom went through was the driving force behind me going into dentistry—a decision I made my senior year in high school. She not only had to deal with chronic discomfort, but there were a lot of psychological issues involved in going to the dentist so often. I was deeply inspired to help people just like her to "slay the dragons of fear" so that going to the dentist wasn't such an ordeal. In my mind, it became my destiny.

Unfortunately, that wasn't the end of the story.

Fast-forward about eight years. Her dental problems had returned in the back of her mouth, with a vengeance. Many of the improvements that had been made were in great jeopardy.

Though she didn't take the best care of her mouth, eating too many of her beloved Mounds candy bars and leaving the bathroom drawer full of unused floss, the biggest part of the problem was that she did not get the right coaching on how to prevent the problems in her mouth.

She was devastated about the prospect of facing a new battle to save her teeth. To make matters worse, this was happening while my dad was trying to help me pay for dental school. As he'd say, "Guess we all will have to work a little harder." He was truly a saint dressed as a workaholic.

Over the course of her life, my mom had to have her mouth essentially remade four times. It seemed like she was always going to the dentist.

Shortly after graduating from Emory Dental School, I sat down with her while she was recovering from having a radical mastectomy to treat breast cancer. Though her life could have been in jeopardy, she talked often about "the gerbil wheel of dentistry" and how hard it was to keep her mouth healthy, while my dad was having to pay for her treatment over and over again. Her downward spiral was heartbreaking. On that spring day in 1986, she made me promise to *never* let anyone go through what she experienced—to be the best dentist I could be and be the best advocate possible for my patients.

It has been my solemn mission ever since to keep the promise I made to her.

Today, I have a thriving practice that is committed to excellence in cosmetic dentistry and wellness. I have spent my years since dental school continuously learning, improving, and bringing into my practice new tools and techniques, and for the last twenty years I have been asked to lecture around the world on the latest advances in dentistry. My goal is to help dentists to see the value of doing a job right, because I've seen too many patients whose procedures have failed. Too often, patients are even traveling for what they believe is a better price. While they may end up in the chair of a dentist who seems to have the best intentions, they are ultimately paying for treatment from someone who is not committed to excellence or who is reaching far beyond his or her capabilities.

I've poured my heart and soul into making dentistry a quest to "do it right." I'm very blessed that people have entrusted me all these many years to do that, and I want to see that legacy continue.

All these years, I've wanted patients to have not only a beautiful and believable smile, but also to bring joy to everyone for a long time by having them always love their appearance and how healthy their mouth feels.

A Love of Education

Since I didn't want to spend four years in undergraduate school—I didn't want my parents to have to spend any more money than they had to—I crushed through college to get into dental school early. Receiving a Phi Beta Kappa award as a junior made it hard to turn me down. I turned twenty-one the day before I entered dental school, and I found myself working with people twice my age. Interestingly, many of my classmates nicknamed me "Rookie" because I was so young.

Very early on, I learned that dental school only teaches what is needed to pass the board and some crucial skills to have once school is over. But the real learning in dentistry comes after that. After graduating from Emory University Dental School in 1983, I participated in a General Practice Residency program at the Veteran's Administration Medical Center in New Orleans, and then performed cosmetic material research at Louisiana State University School of Dentistry. Today, I am accredited by the American Academy of Cosmetic Dentistry (AACD) and am a longtime member, working my up through the organization to become president from 2010 to 2011. I also founded the Georgia Academy of Cosmetic Dentistry, and I've pursued additional education and training through the Kois Center, American Academy of Implant Dentistry, the Academy of Laser Dentistry, and the Pankey Institute.

Over the years, I've been fortunate to have great mentors, including a man considered to be the father of cosmetic dentistry, Dr. Ronald Goldstein—learning dentistry from Dr. Goldstein is to my profession what learning how to hit a ball from Babe Ruth is to baseball.

Since graduating, I've continued to take far more than the required level of continuing education and give a dozen or more lectures each year—to staff and to other dental professionals—inspiring them and forcing me to continually raise my game. I really like seeing the light bulb go on for other dental professionals. That creates a ripple effect that helps patients get better treatment, but also helps dentists enjoy their practice. It helps them to avoid the steep learning curve that used to exist because of less training and fewer materials and technologies available to the industry. Those technologies—lasers, implants, digital scans and models, and more—allow us to stay at the forefront of this ever-evolving industry. While adding technologies to my practice has allowed for a broader range of experience and capabilities, I also know when to collaborate with other professionals to ensure a patient has the best experience, and best outcomes, they can have.

An Oasis for Patients

Having seen what my mom and what many of patients have been through, I have made sure from day one that my practice is an "oasis" for patients who haven't been treated properly, or who are fearful of going to the dentist. People don't deserve to be abused or treated harshly while in the dentist's chair, regardless of the condition of their mouth. Everyone deserves a healthy, beautiful smile.

My team and I hear some mind-boggling stories about how patients have been treated in other practices, and I tend to believe many of them because of what I see on their x-rays and other tests. Often, what they really need is the right guidance, the right strategies to have a much better chance at having a mouth like mine. You see, even though my mom—and my dad—did not have healthy mouths, I'm the opposite. I have not had a filling in my mouth since I was six years old. The difference? I had a great dentist who taught me preventive dentistry. Plus, my dad also swore when I had five small cavities at age six that those would be last cavities ever in my mouth—and that kind of vow coming from my dad, a big, imposing man (built like Tony Soprano and talked like Clint Eastwood), pretty much scared me into having a healthy mouth for life. Fortunately, the dentist was able to preserve a lot of tooth structure when filling those early cavities, so my teeth have remained strong all these years.

What's also different about my practice is how we look beyond the surface—literally. When we see problems in the mouth, we not only want to repair the damage, we want to *find out what's causing the damage*. We want to understand the risk factors that patients have that may be causing bad habits, or poor functionality, or why there is so much wear and tear. In the chapters ahead, I'll discuss some of these factors to help you see how cavities, broken teeth, and other problems in the mouth may be the result of your health or your environment.

There are so many variables involved in correcting problems and risk factors in the mouth that everything must be taken into account when determining treatment—like pieces of a puzzle. I

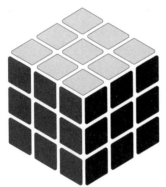

think of each patient's treatment like solving a Rubik's Cube color by color, a concept I learned from one of my mentors, Dr. John Kois, in Seattle, Washington—each patient's risk factors must be solved with a customized treatment plan to create a long-term, stable mouth. As a result, we commonly have patients comment that they knew their smile would be improved, but they did not realize how much the treatment would improve their health and bite overall. In the chapters ahead, I'll share some of these stories with you. In some cases, I've changed the patient's name to protect their privacy.

This book is for anyone who wants to improve their smile for health reasons, to build confidence, or whether they simply want to be happier with the person they see in the mirror. I want to help you understand the importance of a better smile and why it pays to do it right the first time. Furthermore, I want you to see what it means to get a return on your investment.

Just as importantly, I also hope what you will take away from this book is an idea of how to care for yourself every day; a comprehensive understanding of the cosmetic dentistry options available, if and when you would need them; and a desire to improve your smile and your entire world.

THE IMPORTANCE OF A GREAT SMILE

osmetic dentistry covers a wide range of treatment options, from simple whitening procedures to full-mouth reconstruction. Without a real understanding of the value of cosmetic dentistry, many people often put off having a dentist look inside their mouth and come up solutions. However, waiting longer can sometimes make treatment even more challenging.

That was part of the issue with Tracy. The first time Tracy came to see me, she was unhappy with the way her teeth looked. They were yellow and worn down because she had major bite issues. She also had deficiencies in her enamel—the result of genetics—which had weakened her teeth and bone. In addition, she wanted a smile that she could be proud of, so we put together a treatment plan that would involve pretty extensive work, but would allow us to strengthen the foundation of her mouth along with many of her teeth.

Unfortunately, she decided that the plan was not within her budget, so she sought out less-costly treatment from other dentists and settled on one out of town that a family member recommended. With nothing in the way of a blueprint, he gave her a new smile with a row of crowns that were bulky and too uniform to look like the real thing. They looked like she had a row of Chiclets gum instead of teeth.

By the time she came back to see me, Tracy was beside herself because she had invested so much in her smile, and it still wasn't something she was proud to see in the mirror. In fact, the next time I saw Tracy, her gums were inflamed and her bite was worse than ever and painful. Plus, when we took x-rays, we could see that a lot of the crowns were not sealed properly, which meant she was destined for some real problems with bacteria and breakage.

Unfortunately, we had to start from scratch with Tracy because we were unable to obtain any of her information from the dentist who had treated her. We ultimately did what equated to an "extreme makeover" on Tracy. We had to remove all her crowns to treat her for a bacteria avalanche that had begun, straighten her bite while she wore prototype crowns, and then place new, customized-to-her, permanent crowns on her teeth.

Since she had already been burned with the previous treatment, she was very particular with the plan we put together for her. But in the end, she got exactly what she wanted—a smile that she was proud to show to the world.

Tracy's treatment has lasted as well. Since her treatment ended in 2008, I've seen her for regular cleanings and some minor maintenance. But all in all, since her care has been completed, she's lived her life as a working mother with a much happier smile and healthier mouth.

"You get what you pay for! After all I have been through, I am blessed that Dr. Flax is a great dentist with integrity. Thankfully, I have always trusted his abilities to serve my needs and solve my

problems successfully. What a huge bonus that he is also very considerate and compassionate."
—*Tracy*

See Tracy's progress in the before and after photo section.

Cosmetic Dentistry—
Start with the Low-Hanging Fruit

Quite often, people put off addressing problems in their mouth that can be fixed with cosmetic dentistry, because they don't understand just what cosmetic dentistry is about. Not everyone has to go through what Tracy did to enjoy the effects of cosmetic dentistry. Sometimes very simple procedures like whitening, bonding, and contouring can make a big difference in having a great smile—what I call the "low-hanging fruit." It all depends on the patient and their needs.

Everyone is different. Some patients are like Tracy and need a full-mouth reconstruction. Many may need the conservative "low-hanging fruit." Others need procedures to restore the function to their mouth before we can finish up with cosmetics; these patients might have severe wear and need teeth built up, or they might have some crowding and need their teeth straightened, or they may even be missing one or more teeth that need to be replaced.

There's no one-size-fits-all for every patient, which is what you'll find with a lot of practices—they just plug in a solution without trying to preserve any existing, healthy teeth.

If you were to compare what I'm saying to plastic surgery, it would be a little like comparing a Botox procedure to a full-blown facelift. Sometimes, with cosmetic dentistry, just a few nips and tucks—whitening or bonding and shaping—is all it takes to refresh and rejuvenate your smile. I'll talk about the types of procedures that we do at my practice in the chapters ahead.

Too many people put off having a cosmetic dentist look at their mouth because they think it's too expensive or they're beyond help. But, very often, all it takes is a little strategy and some very predictable procedures to give you the smile you've been longing for.

For now, let me share with you a few reasons why you should consider cosmetic dentistry today, rather than waiting.

A Great Smile:
The Window to the Soul

When you smile, it allows people to see that joy and confidence that exists inside of you. If you have a great sense of humor, if you love to laugh, you have to have a smile that is ideal for showing that side of you to the world.

But I've had many patients that have kept that personality bottled up inside. Why? Because they're so embarrassed by their teeth that they never open their mouth and show the world their smile. They may see or hear something they think is really funny, but they refuse to show their smile because they think it makes them look bad. Everyone wants to look good, and teeth are a big part of how a person appears on the outside. A bright, shiny smile can dazzle people from across the room.

A number of studies have found that a beautiful smile can make you appear to be more attractive, and, according to research by Beall Research & Training of Chicago, your smile can even make you appear smarter, more interesting, and even successful and wealthy.[1]

When the American Academy of Cosmetic Dentistry (AACD) had an independent study conducted, the results were eye opening.

---

1   "Can a New Smile Make You Appear More Successful and Intelligent?" American Academy of Cosmetic Dentistry, Consumer Studies news release, accessed February 4, 2019, https://aacd.com/surveys.

Adults in the study were shown photos of people who had undergone cosmetic dentistry. The respondents were not told they were judging a person's smile; instead, they were asked to judge the people in the photos on certain characteristics, including attractiveness, intelligence, happiness, career success, friendliness, kindness, wealth, and whether they would be popular with the opposite sex.[2] Here are findings from this and other studies:

A confidence booster. A flawed smile was perceived to be a sign of less confidence, according to participants in an AACD survey. Twenty-five percent said that's what they saw in an imperfect smile compared to someone with what they viewed as "perfect" teeth.[3]

A career booster. Nearly all Americans in an AACD study (99.7 percent) believed that a smile was an important asset. Some 74 percent thought an unattractive smile could potentially hurt a person's chances at having a successful career.[4]

A more appealing feature to the opposite sex. Ninety-six percent of respondents to an AACD study thought an attractive smile made a person more appealing to members of the opposite sex.[5] Another study also supports the latter finding: a Harris Interactive survey of more than two thousand adults found that nearly three quarters of them (74 percent) prefer to kiss someone with a nice smile over someone with crooked

---

2   Ibid.

3   "A Picture Perfect Smile: The Secret to Attractiveness at Any Age," American Academy of Cosmetic Dentistry, Consumer Studies news release, accessed February 4, 2019, https://aacd.com/surveys.

4   Ibid.

5   "Can a New Smile Make You Appear More Successful and Intelligent?" op. cit.

teeth, and 18 percent of those surveyed through that an imperfect smile was keeping them from finding a mate.[6]

A most memorable feature. When asked about smiles in the photos, respondents to an AACD study said that they most remembered aspects like tooth color, straightness, cleanliness, and sparkle, and that traits like missing or crooked teeth, visible decay, and stains made a smile unattractive.[7] When asked about memorable features, nearly half of participants (48 percent) in another study said the smile was what they remembered most when meeting someone for the first time—more than what a person said, what they were wearing, or their scent.[8]

A feature to improve. When asked about their own smiles, most people in an AACD study said that "whiter and brighter teeth" was the one thing they would like to improve.[9]

An asset when aging. Nearly half (around 45 percent) of participants in an AACD study said a smile is a person's most attractive feature as a person ages, more so than the body (10 percent), hair (6 percent) or legs (5 percent). More than half of the people age fifty or over said that a smile was the most enduring feature as a person ages. Even in younger generations, 39 percent of eighteen- to forty-nine-year-olds found a smile to be a long-term attractive feature.[10]

---

6   "For Today's Singles, the Secret to a Better Love Life May Be a Better Smile," *PRNewswire*, September 9, 2013, accessed February 5, 2019, www.prnewswire.com/news-releases/for-todays-singles-the-secret-to-a-better-love-life-may-be-a-better-smile-222947031.html.

7   "Can a New Smile Make You Appear More Successful and Intelligent?" op. cit.

8   "A Picture Perfect Smile: The Secret to Attractiveness at Any Age," op. cit.

9   "Can a New Smile Make You Appear More Successful and Intelligent?" op. cit.

10 "A Picture Perfect Smile: The Secret to Attractiveness at Any Age," op. cit.

An even greater portion of the people surveyed felt that spending money to have a youthful smile was well worth the investment. Some 84 percent of women and 75 percent of men said they would be willing to invest in treatment for a younger smile, and people aged thirty to thirty-nine were more willing to do so: 88 percent of the people in this age group said they would spend money to improve their looks.[11] Sixty-two percent of people surveyed said they would spend money to improve the quality of their teeth.

There you have it:

- **more confidence**
- **more approachable**
- **sexier**
- **higher self-esteem**

That's what people think when they see a great smile. If your smile is less than ideal, it can really affect how you feel about yourself and how you greet the world.

These surveys prove something that I see every day: A great smile can give you a whole new energy. I see people every day who are embarrassed by their smile. Sometimes, they don't even want to show me their teeth—and I'm the one they've come to for help.

But after we work some magic on them—we take x-rays and photos, create a blueprint, and then apply the new design to a person's smile—it's almost like pulling the string on a talking doll. They're a totally changed person, ready to talk, laugh, and go out into the world.

---

11   Ibid.

First Impressions—
No Longer Just In-Person

With the rise of social media and selfies, everybody wants to look good these days. That's because first impressions no longer happen only face-to-face. In today's digital world, your smile can be seen around the world in an instant. With a just few clicks, virtually millions of people can see you—and your smile—for the first time. That's why a winning smile is so important for helping you make a positive first impression.

People have developed a kind of a defensive pattern so that nobody sees a flaw in their appearance. They'll comb their hair, tilt their head, posture their lips—all in a certain way. That may work for a portrait or even a selfie, but you can't really fake it when meeting people or having conversations—especially considering that 60 percent of the weight of a face is composed of your smile.[12] With your smile being such a prominent feature, it's no wonder it makes such an immediate impact—whether consciously or subconsciously—on the people you meet.

When you can fully express yourself, your whole life changes. Being able to do that opens doors in terms of your overall well-being and happiness. And cosmetic dentistry can make that difference. With a great smile, you can be authentic with your emotions—you can let it all hang out and not have to worry that you're being judged by your appearance.

Too often, I have patients that say, "Just pull them all out." That's how frustrated they are with their teeth and their smile. They're

---

12   "Best Face Forward: Making GREAT First Impressions in a Digital Age," American Academy of Cosmetic Dentistry, Consumer Studies news release, accessed February 4, 2019, https://aacd.com/surveys.

resigned to living with their decaying, disheveled, yellowing teeth, and they're despondent about their appearance. But I don't believe that's the answer. I know the importance of permanent teeth, and we do what we can to save them.

Understanding our patients' needs begins by talking to them about their concerns and what they envision for their ideal smile. It's very illuminating to be able to get into that collaborative mode with patients—they tell me what they want, what they don't want. Many times, what they tell me is they want something that looks natural, that's not going to shock everyone or "glow in the dark." Some people want a whole new image, others want to return their smile to what it was when they were younger. Especially when someone wants to turn back the clock, we ask for a picture of them from when they were younger. We want to see what they're envisioning, whether we can turn back the clock that far or not.

Then there are patients that don't know what they want, they just hate the way they look. With only that information to go on, we start by talking about the color of their teeth and what might be appropriate for them considering the whites of their eyes, skin complexion, hair color, and age.

Depending on those and other factors, we'll look at the shapes of their teeth, the number of teeth showing, the condition and symmetry of their gums. The truth is, we're not going to return a seventy-year-old woman's smile back to what it was in high school, but we can certainly do some things to shave off many years.

Proven: A Healthy Smile
Adds Years to Your Life

In addition to how a smile looks and helps you present yourself, a great smile is a healthy smile. Oral health is just as important as overall wellness—in fact, the two are very connected. Problems in the mouth can signal a problem somewhere else in the body, and when a person's mouth is not healthy, it can actually affect the health of their body.

The mouth is filled with bacteria, most of which is not harmful. These bacteria produce acids, which can be washed away by saliva in the mouth. It's a system of balance that is controlled, in part, by regular brushing and flossing. Good oral hygiene along with the body's natural defenses can keep harmful bacteria in the mouth in check. When those bacteria get out of control because of a lack of proper oral hygiene, or because of reduced saliva from taking certain medications, then you can begin to have problems such as gum disease and tooth decay.

Some diseases can lower the body's defenses, making it easier to develop inflammation in the mouth. That can lead to periodontitis, which is a severe form of gum disease.

Studies have begun to link the inflammation and infection from poor oral health to problems such as heart disease, premature birth, and low birth weights.[13] Links have also been found between conditions such as diabetes—people with uncontrolled blood sugar levels often develop gum disease, and when a person has gum disease, it can be harder to control their diabetes. It's a two-way street.[14] Other

---

13 Mayo Clinic Staff, "Oral Health: A Window to Your Overall Health," *Mayo Clinic*, November 1, 2018, accessed February 5, 2019, www.mayoclinic.org/ healthy-lifestyle/adult-health/in-depth/dental/art-20047475%20--.

14 Ibid.

health problems that can lead to problems in the mouth include Alzheimer's disease, oral cancer, HIV/AIDS, eating disorders, rheumatoid arthritis, and osteoporosis (because of the drugs used to treat it).

HOW CAN I PROTECT MY ORAL HEALTH?

To protect your oral health, practice good oral hygiene every day:

- Brush your teeth at least twice a day with fluoride toothpaste.

- Floss daily.

- Eat a healthy diet and limit between-meal snacks.

- Replace your toothbrush every three to four months, or sooner if bristles are frayed.

- Schedule regular dental checkups and cleanings.

- Avoid tobacco use.

Advantages of Having a Healthy Smile

A healthy smile allows you to eat healthier foods. Stronger teeth and bone let you chew with more power. That's what's needed to grind and shred food. One of my more challenging cases involved a young woman with some congenital issues that required her to have major surgeries just to get the foundation of her mouth in a condition where we could begin to build teeth. Without having teeth that were strong enough to chew healthy food, she had begun gaining a lot of weight—and she was only twenty-two years old.

A lack of healthy teeth can create so many consequences in your life that they can snowball:

- You can't smile.

- Then you can't chew.

- Your health starts deteriorating.

- You may become overweight and diabetic.

- You can't sleep well.

- That makes you lethargic and keeps you from competing in the business world or enjoying a social life.

Your life just goes down a rabbit hole.

If your bite doesn't fit together—the surfaces don't fit together or the teeth aren't aligned properly—then you can't chew efficiently, forcing you to favor one side or one area of the mouth. You may find yourself in a lot of pain, and you won't know why. That happened to one of my patients. She was frustrated because she had strong teeth, but had undergone several root canals. "I don't know if I really needed those root canals," she told me. "It's just like my bite just hasn't been right." I'll talk more about the bite in chapter 3.

Missing teeth can also lead to bone loss over time. If adjacent teeth have to work harder because of a missing tooth, that overload can start to cause breakdown. Implants, which substitute for missing teeth, can be just as damaging since they fuse to the bone. Without any sort of shock absorber, the bite can become more sensitive in that area. In my practice, I place implants for teeth that are beyond health, and I'll talk more about that in chapter 8.

When your teeth are stable, you don't have to worry about emergencies. You don't suddenly have to call up the dentist and take a day off work to have swelling in your mouth or an abscessed gum treated. A patient came to see me one time to help with a tooth she had glued back into her mouth—she was going to be in a professional debate that day, and was so desperate when her tooth dislodged that morning that she just glued it back in. By the time she came to see me, her mouth was in such a state that she needed a full reconstruction. Now, she's a different person—and wouldn't think of using Super Glue in her mouth.

Tracy—A Happy, Healthy, Worry-Free Mouth

For Tracy, the road to a healthy mouth began after she first took a detour. Today, she has a mouth that is no longer painful, and no longer an overwhelming part of her everyday concerns as a working mother.

The moral of the story is this: A stable, healthy mouth gives you peace of mind. You don't have to worry about the pain—physical or financial. You don't have to deal with discomfort. You don't have to miss work or resort to desperate measures. You're able to eat and enjoy life—and smile about it.

In the upcoming chapters, I'll talk about different cosmetic procedures that can help you have a smile you'll be proud to wear and that will help you have a happier life.

For now, let's look at the most conservative cosmetic dentistry option—teeth whitening.

SMILE ON!

What you can do now to get started:

- Research dentists who are accredited with the AACD.

- Brush and floss properly to keep stains off teeth and keep food from between teeth.

- Schedule a professional dental cleaning and checkup.

CHAPTER 2

WHITENING: TRUTH OR CONSEQUENCES

When Elaine came to see me to make her smile whiter and brighter, the condition of her mouth seemed hopeless. She had multiple teeth that were so broken down that the only choice was to replace them with implants. She was pretty frustrated with dentists as a whole by that point, because a lot of promises had been made to her but few had been delivered.

Seeing how distressed she was, we told her, "Let's start with some baby steps." We knew that, in order to get Elaine to the finish line of her treatment, we needed to build some trust with her.

Unfortunately, those baby steps began by removing teeth that were beyond repair. Then we worked on getting her mouth healthier so that it would hold the implants in the bone. After we placed the implants and they were integrating into the bone, she decided she wanted more than just the missing teeth replaced. She wanted all of her teeth to be straight as well—she had become comfortable with us and with her treatment. We put her in Invisalign clear aligners to straighten the rest of her teeth.

Then, before placing the crowns on the implants, Elaine decided to "go the distance"—she wanted all of her teeth to be whiter. We performed a conservative and comfortable whitening procedure and placed the implant crowns, and now she can smile and eat with confidence—and to show her true self. She has a great sense of humor with a great laugh, and now readily shares both with anyone she meets.

For Elaine, who wanted to look natural, be healthy, and have peace of mind in knowing that the problems of her mouth were solved, we were able to complete the journey by building trust and keeping our promise—giving her the smile she wanted.

Before I met Dr. Flax, several unfortunate experiences had left me with a strong aversion to visiting any dentist anywhere. However, I eventually developed a set of conditions—including fractured molars, infections, and misaligned front teeth—that needed professional attention. At Flax Dental, I finally found a practice that respected my questions and concerns. Over approximately thirty months, Dr. Flax and his team worked with me to implement a step-by-step plan to address both the health and appearance of what Dr. Flax calls "my smile." That plan incorporated dental implants, filling repair, Invisalign therapy, and a whitening program, as well as regular cleanings. The end result has been not only the restoration of my smile, but a renewed confidence in dental care, knowing that Dr. Flax offers a level of compassionate professionalism and technical expertise that I can trust without hesitation.

—Elaine
patient.

See Elaine's progress in the before and after photo section

Hits—and Myths—About Whitening

There is a lot of misunderstanding about whitening teeth. Here are some of the more common truths and misconceptions.

Cosmetic dentistry does not stain. True and false. It depends on the material used. Porcelain does not stain, yet it also cannot be whitened. Once placed in the mouth, crowns or bridges made of porcelain remain their original color. With Elaine, the challenge was to whiten her existing teeth to match the implant-supported crowns that were replacing missing teeth.

Crowding and crevices are harder to whiten. It's true that crowded teeth can create overlapped areas or crevices that are difficult to reach with over-the-counter strips. But professional whitening that is brushed on or that comes with customized trays and clinical gel can reach places in between teeth. However, when a tooth is rotated, the flat surface of a tooth does not face outward. Sides of teeth create a more deflective type of light, whereas the wide, flat surface of a tooth reflects more light, making it look whiter.

Imagine the folds of a window drape or hanging curtain: where the curtain folds in toward the wall or window, the cloth is darker, it's in shadow; where the folds curl outward, into the room, the material is lighter, brighter, and may even have a sheen.

Elaine saw how her turned teeth were less beautiful—because they did not reflect the light—which is one reason why she wanted them straightened before whitening.

Genetics, medications discolor teeth. Yes, genetics and medications taken during growth and development as a child can discolor teeth. These stains typically cannot be whitened by over-the-counter or in-office procedures, but there are other cosmetic dentistry procedures that can create a brighter smile (such as bonding or veneers, which I will talk about in the chapters ahead).

Aging teeth cannot be whitened. Not true. Older teeth have typically lost some of the enamel outer layer, leading to duller-looking teeth. Sometimes, that's because of too much acidity in a person's diet or from the stomach as a result of a health problem or because of purposeful purging due to bulimia. Friction from a lifetime of chewing can also cause wear in the form of brown lines, craze lines, and cracks in the teeth. Over time, bacteria and stains get into those cracks, and the teeth start to show discoloration as a result. But teeth can be whitened at any age.

Flexing teeth can cause discoloration. Yes, this is true. When a person's bite is off, it can cause teeth to flex. That can create concave or yellow areas near the gumline where the root begins to show through. Known as an **abfraction**, these areas can worsen with aggressive toothbrushing or abrasive toothpastes. When these areas begin to decay, brown stains begin to appear on the teeth or the tooth becomes sensitive—especially to whitening products. To avoid such complications, a tooth with an abfraction should be repaired.

Professional versus Do-It-Yourself Whitening

Whitening used to be an uncomfortable and laborious process. Known as **in-office bleaching** in the 1970s and 1980s, the procedure involved placing a rubber covering over each tooth as a way of protecting the gums prior to placing very strong bleaching gels that were activated by a strong heat lamp. Usually one arch was "bleached" at each session. Ugh.

Then, in the late 1980s, a new technique was discovered. Up to that point, dentists often used peroxide to treat their patients' gums, with a side effect being whiter teeth. By adding peroxide to a gel inside a tray applied to the teeth, whitening became easier and affordable for anyone who wanted a brighter smile. Amen!

It's preferable to whiten a healthy mouth, so the process starts by determining whether there are any issues that must be addressed. We want to know whether all the teeth fit together well, whether there is significant crowding, or whether there are cracks or other issues with the teeth. If there is decay under a crown, or an open cavity, whitening gel could cause significant discomfort—that opening in a tooth makes an easier path to the nerve of the tooth. We also look for health issues, such as gum recession; often, someone whose gums have receded may already have teeth that are sensitive to temperatures.

Whitening is available in in-office and we have some take-home choices. Patients who want quick results or who don't have the time or discipline to whiten their teeth with take-home trays typically opt for the in-office procedures.

Power (or accelerated) in-office whitening is an updated version of the one from decades ago and allows for both upper and lower teeth to be done simultaneously. After a protective resin is placed along the gums (in lieu of the rubber covering), a special gel is brushed onto each natural tooth. A light is then applied to the teeth to accelerate the effect of the whitening gel. This procedure is monitored and controlled by the dental professional, and it produces some very nice, white teeth within a few hours. Please avoid the "mall versions" of this technique because there is usually a lack of training for the technician.

Take-home whitening includes having custom-fitted trays made. By having trays made to fit your teeth, you can avoid irritation of the gums and any areas where tooth roots are exposed because of receding gums. The take-home trays are made by scanning the teeth with a "wand" to produce a digital model of the teeth that is used to print out a three-dimensional model. That model is used to create the customized whitening trays. I'll talk more about this advanced mode of modeling in the chapters ahead.

Whitening done by a cosmetic dentist's office comes with customized instructions. Since there are several strengths of whitening available, patients need to understand their choices and how to use the materials supplied to get the maximum result while being comfortable and having some control of the process.

Some patients opt for both in-office and take-home. They start out with the in-office procedure that puts their whitening on the fast track. Then, they'll have customized trays made and finish up their whitening with take-home gel.

The customized, take-home whitening trays are better than over-the-counter solutions. The trays are filled with a gel that works on all the surfaces of each tooth, not just the surfaces that are flat. Since the trays are customized, and the whitening solution is a gel, it is able to get in between the teeth and into the different curves and undercuts of each tooth.

The trays are made to last, but gel supplies must be replenished now and then. It's best to whiten after having teeth professionally cleaned because the porosities of the teeth have been cleansed, which means there's a greater chance of the whitener being able to penetrate.

The whitening products used by cosmetic dentists are carefully tested and researched for stability and effectiveness. They tend to be safer for the enamel. Plus, they tend to provide longer-lasting results, depending on home dental care and personal habits. Smoking or chewing tobacco, drinking naturally staining beverages such as red wine and coffee, or using drugs are all habits that can damage and discolor teeth.

Over-the-Counter Whitening Options

Over-the-counter whitening options don't match up to professional whitening. Whitening strips, for instance, can't adapt to all the curvatures of the teeth, so you don't get an intimate whitening. If you have gaps in your teeth, using a strip would be a little like trying to span a joint with a Band-Aid—it won't fully cover the area you're trying to whiten.

Some of the early whitening toothpastes advertised that they made teeth "appear" whiter—the teeth appeared whiter because the chemistry of these products reddened the gums. Just like putting a new frame on a picture can change how it looks to the eye, so making the gums redder was basically reframing the teeth and making them "appear" to be whiter.

Many over-the-counter toothpastes that claim to whiten teeth will clean off the stains, but, in doing so, they also take away some of the enamel. While the ingredient baking soda is safe and effective for removing stains, the particle size of many commercially produced, over-the-counter toothpastes makes them too abrasive for teeth. The following page has many recommended toothpastes that are safe and effective.

Abrasiveness Index of Common Toothpastes

Recommended by Dr. Flax

TOOTHPASTE	RDA VALUE
Oral Neutralizing Gel	4
Straight Baking Soda	7
Arm & Hammer Tooth Powder	8
CTx4 gel	17
Arm & Hammer Dental Care	35
Oxyfresh	45
Tom's of Maine Sensitive	49
Arm & Hammer Peroxicare	49
Rembrandt Original	53
CloSYS	53
Tom's of Maine Children's	57
Colgate Sensitive Enamel Protect	67
Colgate Regular	68
Colgate Clean Mint	70
Sensodyne	79
Aim	80
Colgate Sensitive Max Strength	83
Aquafresh Sensitive	91
Tom's of Maine Regular	93
Crest Regular	95
Mentadent	103
Sensodyne Extra Whitening	104
Colgate Platinum	106
Crest Sensitivity	107
Colgate Herbal	110
Aquafresh Whitening	113
Arm & Hammer Tarter Control	117
Arm & Hammer Advance White Gel	117
Closeup with Baking Soda	120
Colgate Whitening	124
Crest Extra Whitening	130
Ultra Brite	133
Crest MultiCare Whitening	144
Colgate Baking Soda Whitening	145
Pepsodent	150
Colgate Tarter Control	165
Colgate Total Gum Defense	185
Colgate 2-1 Tarter Control/White	200
FDA RECOMMENDED LIMIT	**200**
ADA RECOMMENDED LIMIT	**250**

The RDA table:
0-70 = low abrasive
70-100 = medium abrasive
100-150 = highly abrasive
150-250= harmful limit

Source: https://www.healingteethnaturally.com/toothpaste-abrasiveness-index.html

There are also products on the market with very low pH, meaning they're very acidic. These can etch the outside of the tooth, creating the appearance that the teeth are whiter. What they actually do, however, is clean off some of the natural colors of the tooth and, in the process, make the tooth more porous. That makes it more prone to bacteria and more sensitive to temperature. See chapter 9 for more details on how acidity and pH levels can affect your teeth.

Home Remedies—Some Good, Some Bad, Some Really Ugly

There are a number of home remedies that people like to use for whitening teeth. Here are some that work—and some that don't.

Baking soda. Yes, baking soda is an abrasive. But it is gentle enough to remove some stains without harming teeth.

Whitening toothpastes are usually too abrasive on the enamel.

Charcoal is often promoted as a natural tooth whitener. The best way to use that particular product? Don't. Charcoal is too abrasive for teeth.

A study published in *The Journal of the American Dental Association* found no real evidence to support claims that charcoal is effective as a toothpaste, and that it may even cause harm.[15] In an article reporting the study, American Dental Association spokesperson Ada Cooper, DDS, said, "Charcoal is recognized as an abrasive mineral to teeth and gums. Using

---

15   John K. Brooks, Nasir Bashirelahi, and Mark A. Reynolds, "Charcoal and Charcoal-Based Dentifrices: A Literature Review," *JADA: The Journal of the American Dental Association* 148, no. 9 (September 2017): 661–70, https://doi.org/10.1016/j.adaj.2017.05.001.

materials that are too abrasive can actually make your teeth look more yellow, because it can wear away the tooth's enamel and expose the softer, yellower layer called dentin."[16]

Hard toothbrushes abrade the teeth and gums.

Wearing brighter red lipstick. Just as clothing can help hide some flaws, red-based lipsticks can give the illusion of whiter teeth.

Whitening mouth rinses are ineffective. Many of these contain a diluted solution of peroxide, but they are not designed to remain on the teeth long enough to work well as a whitener.

Rinsing with peroxide may freshen your mouth a bit, and it's very useful for treating gums because it breaks down many of the harmful enzymes that cause breakdown in the mouth. However, overuse of peroxide can also upset the balance in the mouth. While it's not the most effective whitener (again, because it doesn't remain on the teeth), for those patients that like using it to cleanse their mouth, we recommend that it be diluted either by combining it with baking soda as a toothpaste, or by adding it to the water in an irrigator (like a Waterpik).

On the White Track

So, what are some of the more common reasons that people choose to whiten their teeth?

---

16 Emily Shiffer, "What Dentists Want You to Know About Those Charcoal Tooth-pastes That Promise Whiter Teeth," *PopSugar*, March 7, 2019, as quoted in *Yahoo Finance*, accessed March 25, 2019, https://finance.yahoo.com/news/dentists-want-know-those-charcoal-193034027.html.

With cosmetic dentistry. Whitening is a good finishing touch when you are improving your smile with cosmetic dentistry such as veneers, bonding, and crowns.

After orthodontics. Whitening can give orthodontic treatment a little something extra. At my office, we provide ongoing dental care during and after orthodontic treatment, so we like to give straightened teeth that added sparkle with whitening. We have several different whiteners available and prescribe the one that's best for each patient's specific needs.

For a special event. For many people, whitening is part of planning for a special event such as a job interview, wedding, or class reunion.

As a reward. Whitening is a great way to celebrate when you've reached a goal toward self-improvement, such as quitting smoking, losing weight, or graduating.

When you want to feel younger. If you're approaching a milestone birthday or anniversary, a great way to peel back a few years is to take your teeth back a few shades.

In fact, at times, I've seen patients improve their smile and then use that as the starting point for more self-improvement, or even a complete makeover. They'll come back a few months later for a checkup, and they're barely recognizable—they've lost weight, changed their hairstyle, and changed the way they dress.

Whitening—
The Final Step for Elaine

For Elaine, whitening was the last leg of a journey to a healthier smile. After extractions, straightening, and implants, she had regained her smile—and her trust in dentistry—and decided to go the distance by whitening her teeth so that everything matched.

Of course, whitening doesn't solve issues such as chipped or broken teeth, or crowded or crooked teeth. But we have other cosmetic procedures that can help with these issues and improve your smile. Let me start by telling you about straightening, which was one of the treatments that worked very well for Elaine.

SMILE ON!

What you can do now to get started:

- Have a professional dental cleaning.

- Eat fresh fruits and vegetables. Certain fruits, such as strawberries, have some natural abrasiveness to them. Eating these "natural whiteners" can help clean some of the debris off your teeth.

- Talk to a qualified cosmetic dentist.

CHAPTER 3

STRAIGHTENING— LOOKS GREAT AND PRESERVES YOUR TEETH

When David came in for his first appointment, he had chipped front teeth and a lot of crowding. The two issues were related—the crowding caused a lot of friction, which led to all the chips. It's like tires on a car—when they are not aligned, they unevenly wear and tear because of all the friction. When that happens to teeth over twenty-five or thirty years, they can end up with chips like David's.

David wanted to improve his smile, and he wanted a solution that would last a long time. We decided the best treatment for David was ABB—Align, Bleach or brighten, and Bond (not to be confused with the Allman Brothers Band.) A friend of mine, Dr. Tif Qureshi, of Wimpole Street Orthodontic Practice in England and past president of the British Academy of Cosmetic Dentistry, originated and teaches the ABB concept as the best way to help people have a natural, affordable smile that is customized to their needs.

We started David's treatment by straightening his teeth with Invisalign, the big daddy of clear aligner systems. That took six months. We also whitened his teeth and used bonding material to repair the chips and flaws. The final look was ideal for someone who travels the world driving Porsches as a hobby.

> *"The whole office is great. I was amazed seeing the before and after photos of my teeth and my smile. Very satisfied with the entire experience. Dr. Flax and his entire staff are very knowledgeable and professional."*
>
> **—David R.**

See David's progress in the before and after photo section.

Brace Yourself: Straightening Benefits

When the teeth are straight, it's *easier to keep them clean*. It's easier to floss because the surfaces are flatter, and there are fewer crevices where bacteria can cause a buildup of calculus and lead to tooth decay and, over time, unhealthy gums.

Straight teeth also *improve your bite*. Your teeth have peaks and valleys. When everything fits together correctly, the peaks fill the valleys of the opposing teeth—peaks in the upper teeth, for instance, fill valleys in lower teeth. When your teeth are aligned properly, it's much easier to have those peaks and valleys line up. *That reduces or eliminates the friction that can cause wear and tear*, helping to conserve tooth structure and prevent chipping of teeth.

When your bite fits together better, *your jaw muscles also work*

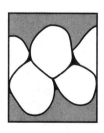

HOW TEETH SHOULD FIT TOGETHER

TRACY

Before:

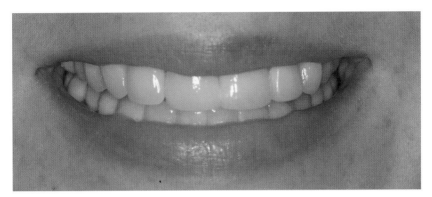

After:

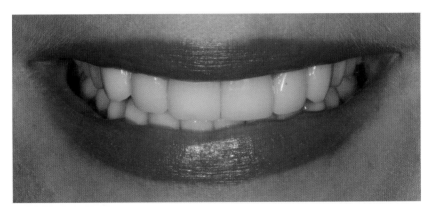

Before and after photos of Tracy from chapter 1, displaying her initial bulky crowns that were not sealed properly. We placed new, customized crowns for her that should last her a lifetime.

ELAINE

Before:

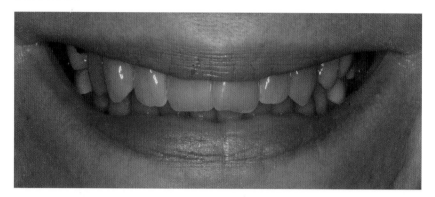

After:

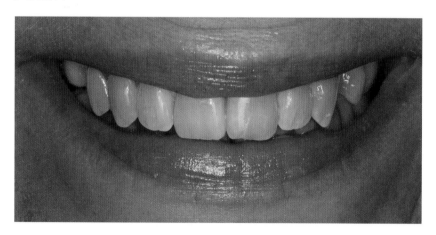

Photos of Elaine from chapter 2, who had multiple broken down teeth that needed to be replaced with implants. We placed implants, straightened them with Invisalign, and then performed a conservative whitening procedure to transform her smile.

DAVID

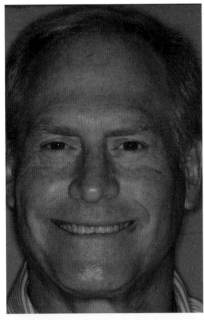

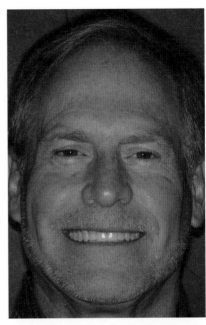

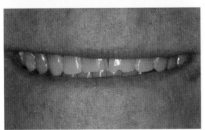

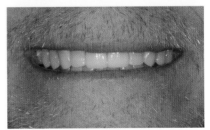

In chapter 3 we talked about David—he had very crowded teeth which led to the front teeth chipping. We decided on the ABB (Align, Bleach or Brighten, and Bond) treatment method popularized by Dr. Tif Qureshi. We aligned his teeth with Invisalign, whitened his teeth, and used bonding material to repair the chips and flaws.

FRANCES

Before:

After:

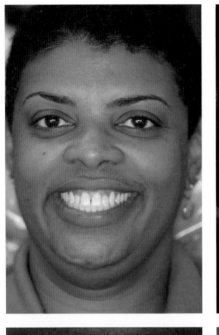

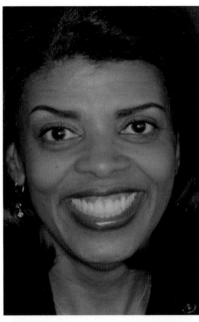

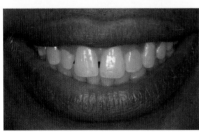

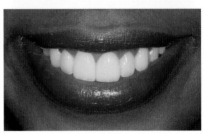

Frances, a chief human resources officer for Gwinnett County Public Schools, came in to fix her big front gap, overbite, uneven teeth, and the discoloration at my office. We used Invisalign and veneers to fix her smile. Read her full story at the front of the book about how her transformation took place!

ANNA

Before: **After:**

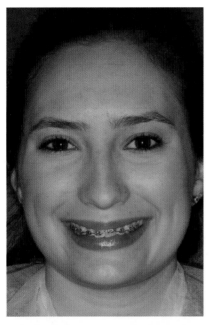
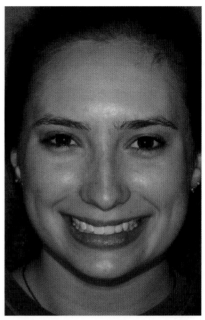

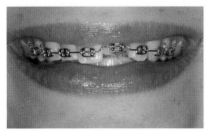
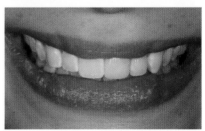

Photos of Anna, discussed in chapter 4, who fell during her senior year in college and traumatized her two front teeth. She received a lot of treatment, including working with an oral surgeon, an orthodontist, and an endodontist. Following those treatments, we helped fix her teeth with bonding.

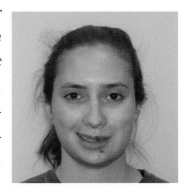

MICHELLE

Before:

After:

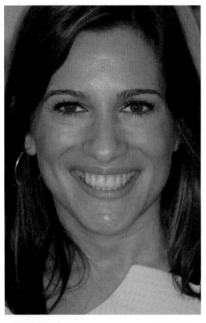
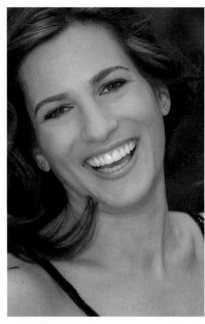

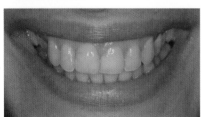
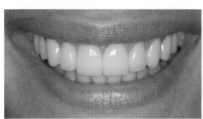

Michelle, from chapter 5, was always told her angled and chipped teeth would require jaw surgery, as she didn't want braces. We used veneers on her ten upper teeth to create an illusion they were straightened, while building volume in her smile. We barely had to remove any tooth structure and only mildly contoured her gums.

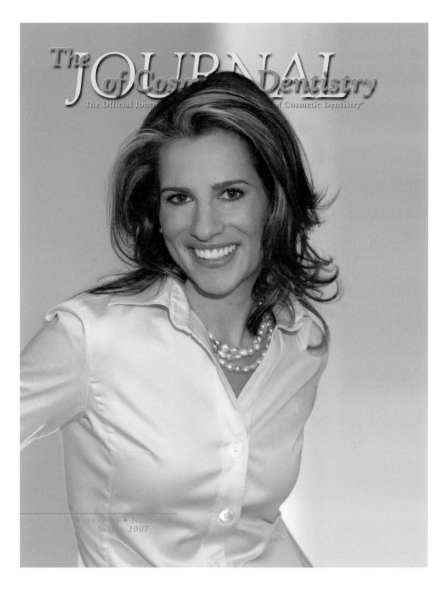

The JOURNAL of Cosmetic Dentistry

The Official Journal of the American Academy of Cosmetic Dentistry

VOLUME 3 • NUMBER
SPRING 2007

Her finished smile is featured quite often in literature and she was featured on a cover of the Journal of Cosmetic Dentistry.

EDI

Before:

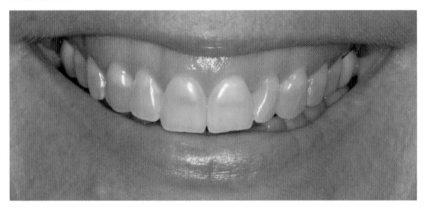

After:

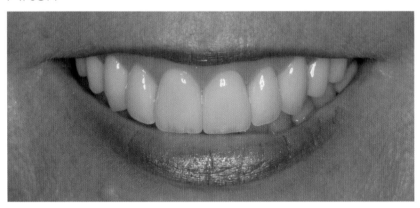

Before and after photos of treatment using veneers assisted by laser gum sculpting.

AMY

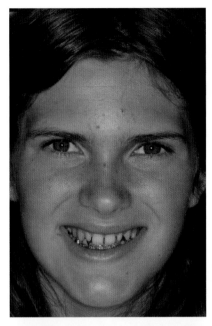
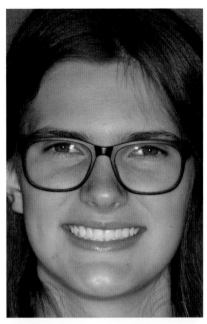
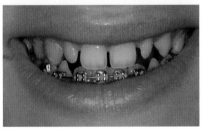
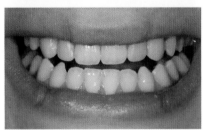

Amy had orthodontic care with a specialist to realign her teeth and correct her bite. This was followed by conservative whitening and bonding to optimize her smile.

HAZEL

Before:

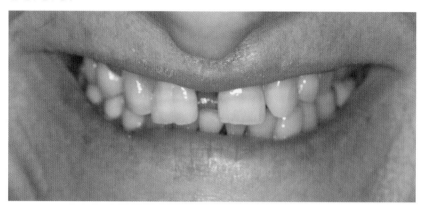

After:

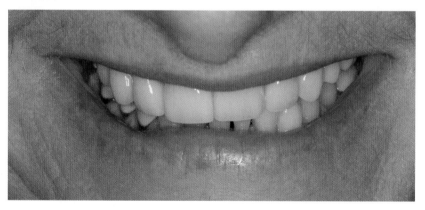

Hazel's before and after photos from chapter 6. We fixed Hazel's smile by using orthodontics to correct the sizable gap in her teeth, and then recontouring her gums to give her a more symmetrical smile.

JANE

Before:

After:

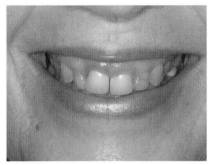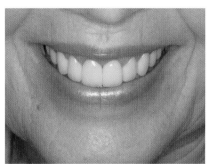

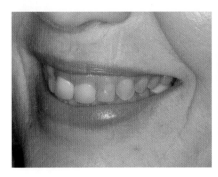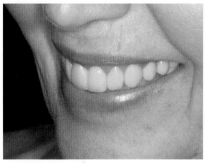

After many years of having a gummy smile and dark teeth, Jane wanted her smile to look great at her son's wedding. Using special smile planning techniques, she had a lasergum lift, new crowns on her front two teeth, and veneers for the adjacent ones. She is now confident and radiant all the time.

ADRIANA

Before:

After:

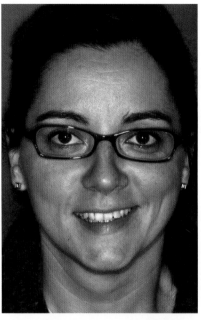
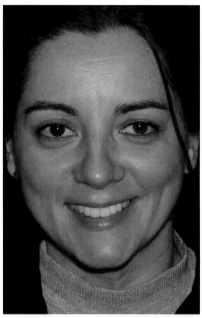
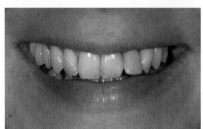
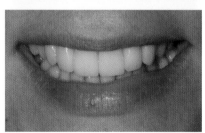

Adriana from chapter 8 always experienced dental anxiety and had bad experiences with dentistry in Eastern Europe. She came to us because an implant that wasn't done right caused an irritation in her gums. She also had broken-down teeth. We saved the implant and placed a few more to fix her smile—and most importantly, she is no longer afraid of the dentist!

"TEETH IN A DAY" PATIENT

Before:

After:

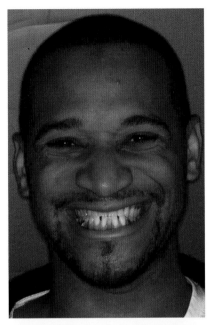
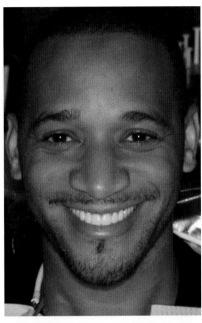
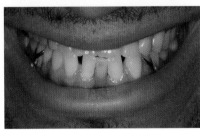
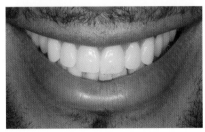

An example of a patient who underwent "Teeth In a Day" treatment, which involves removing the teeth, cleaning up the bone, placing multiple implants, and then placing a one-piece prosthesis on the implants to act as a permanent bridge.

KEVIN

Before: After:

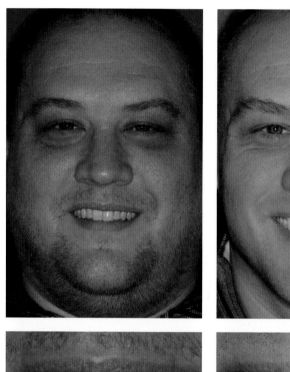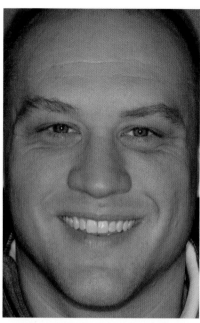

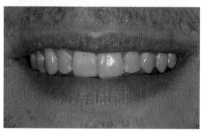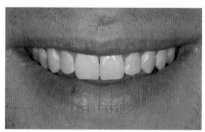

Kevin from chapter 9 came to us with multiple, serious oral health concerns that was also affecting his overall health and wellness. We performed a combination of treatments looking at his gums, his bite, and his teeth. Once Kevin's oral health was improved, the rest of his overall health improved as well—read the full story on Kevin in chapter 9.

ASHLEY

Before:

After:

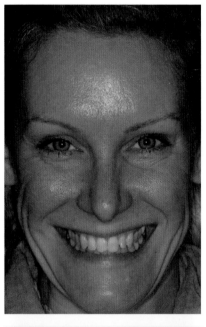
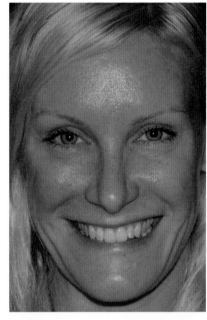

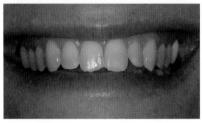
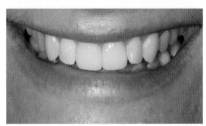

Ashley, who was very fearful (as mentioned in Chapter 10), was able to overcome her fears as we built trust and collaboration—with a little help of sedation as well. Ultimately, she has developed health and confidence with stronger teeth and a new smile.

ANN

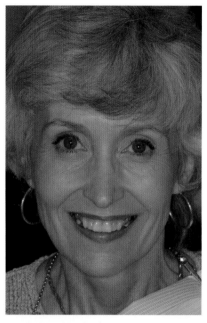

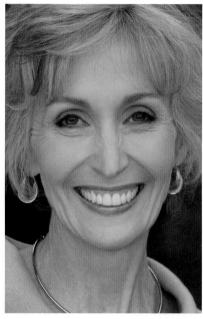

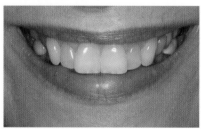

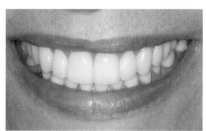

Ann wanted an updated, more youthful appearance. A combination of whitening, veneers, and porcelain crowns gave her a more radiant look and confidence that she was excited to share.

ELIZABETH

Before:

After:

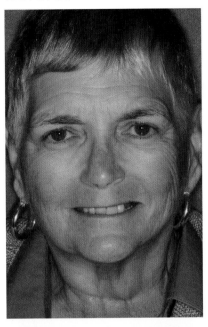
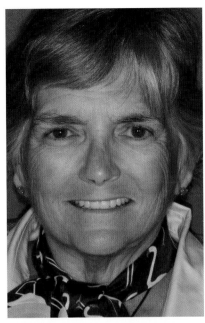

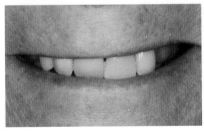
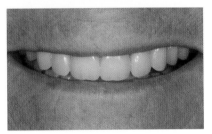

Very fearful and in pain for many years, Elizabeth struggled to find a dental office she could trust. Ultimately, when she found us, many of her teeth and implants were beyond saving. Fortunately, the Teeth in a Day technique have give her the confidence to smile and enjoy food that she had been craving for many years.

RUSSELL

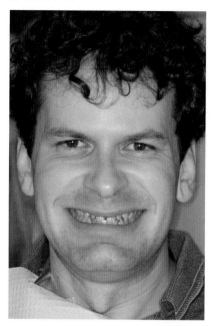 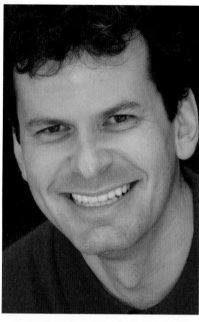

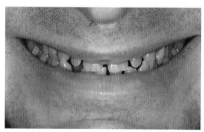 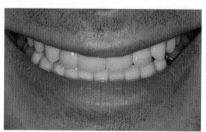

Russell was very frustrated with the "gothic look" of his smile due to his crowded, dark teeth. With detailed smile planning, orthodontics, veneers, and crowns—assisted with a laser gum lift—we were able to give him the smile he had always dreamed of.

KAREN

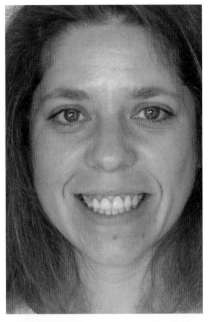
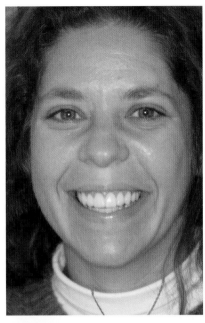

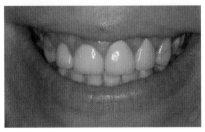
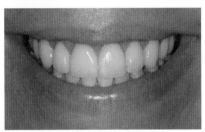

Karen was embarrassed by poor looking crowns that also irritated her gums. Combining laser gum therapy with new crowns, as well as adding veneers, improved the brightness and proportions of the teeth. (Note: the original crowns looked too large because Karen's teeth needed orthodontics to close her teenage spaces. Proper planning has long term implications.)

JOHN

Before:

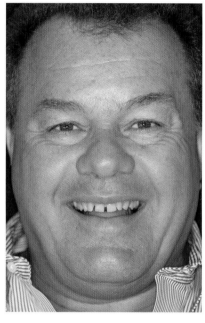

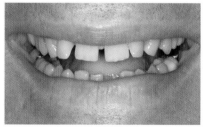

After:

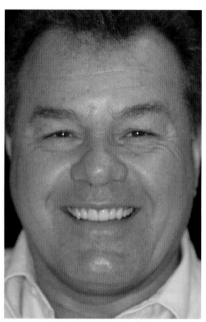

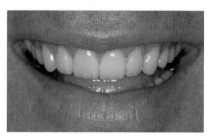

John, who was very anxious about going to the dentist, wanted to close the spaces in his smile, as well as show more back teeth and repair worn front ones. The solution was bite therapy, smile planning, and placing veneers while using oral sedation. He was ecstatic and more confident about his rejuvenated appearance.

better. It's easier to chew different types of food that require jaw power—foods like steak and chicken, fresh vegetables, and fruits.

THE BENEFITS OF STRAIGHT TEETH

- Easier to keep clean

- Improves your bite

- Reduces or eliminates friction

- Less wear and tear

- Jaw muscles work better

KEY POINT: If you allow your teeth to continue to wear down, then it takes more complicated procedures to make the teeth strong and attractive. The more proactive you are, the less-complicated your care has to be. Just like people who exercise are less likely to need tummy tucks, making sure you have a good bite is the best way to preserve your teeth. The longer you procrastinate, the more excuses you make, the less tooth structure and bone you may have to work with. I had a patient who had a problem tooth in the front for years. We tried to help her along the way, but she put off having any real treatment until there was no other option than to replace that tooth with an implant.

Methods for Aligning Teeth

There are several options for aligning teeth: Clear Aligners, Six Month Smiles, traditional braces, or lingual braces.

Aligner Therapy (ClearCorrect and Invisalign). These are the brand names of clear aligner systems, which are a series of plastic trays that are custom fitted to teeth. The trays are changed out over the course of treatment, and each new set of trays moves the teeth closer to the end goal.

Aligners allow us to straighten teeth without the traditional braces system of brackets and wires. With aligners, instead of brackets, small attachments are bonded to the teeth to act like little bumpers for the aligners to push on to move teeth during treatment.

Six Month Smiles. Unlike traditional braces, which are often worn twelve or more months, Six Month Smiles is a procedure that straightens teeth more quickly. This system is designed to straighten the teeth that show during a smile. The treatment uses traditional braces that have tooth-colored brackets and a white wire. In some cases, Six Month Smiles may be used in a hybrid treatment solution; the first few months of treatment uses traditional braces and then the patient is supplied clear aligners for the duration of care.

Traditional braces. When a patient needs extensive orthodontics to correct their bite, traditional braces may be the only option for treatment. In cases where a patient's corrections are very complex and involve a lot of mechanics, we work with select orthodontists to help the patient get back the best function for their mouth. If needed and desired by the patient, we can then follow up by applying the finishing touches to the teeth with a number of functional (bite related) and cosmetic dentistry options.

Lingual braces. These are wires that attach to the back of the front teeth. Lingual braces are often chosen by people who want their teeth straightened, but for whom appearances are very important—high-ranking officials, company leaders, television personalities, and so on.

Accelerated orthodontics. Sometimes crowding is so severe that, to make treatment more efficient, we'll have a periodontist actually cut the bone between the teeth and then move the teeth with the bone—all at the same time. This procedure, known as **corticotomy**, is different than traditional orthodontics, which moves the teeth through a process that changes the bone ahead of a tooth (in the space where the tooth is moving), and then builds bone behind the tooth. If there is an added risk of the bone becoming too thin during traditional orthodontics, then corticotomy is an accelerated and extremely predictable periodontal procedure that can be combined with orthodontics to actually save time when straightening the teeth.

Preparation for Treatment

Several steps must be taken before straightening begins. That includes creating patient records using digital and other technologies. Those digital files are used to communicate with the lab or specialist that fabricates the braces or aligners. Sometimes, a number of treatments must be done to ensure the teeth and gums are healthy before moving forward.

Creating patient records. Evaluation prior to treatment begins with putting together the proper records to determine your exact needs. Those records include digital scanning, photos, videos, and x-rays.

The digital scanning process involves using a wand to create a series of images of your teeth. These images come together in a digital model on the computer screen that allows for your treatment plan to be designed. Virtual smile software can even show you before-and-after views of your smile— you can see what your straightened smile will look like even before treatment begins.

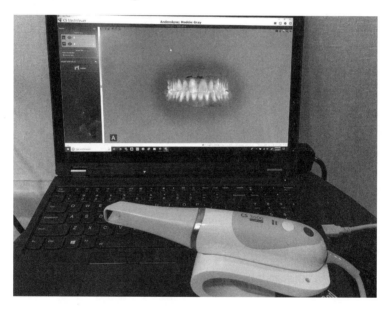

A number of photos and videos are also taken prior to treatment. These may include your teeth and gums and your face from different front and side views—in static and video motion to record speech and bite patterns. These images provide insight into your profile and skeletal relationships— where your mouth is in relation to the rest of your face. For instance, the photographs show if your upper or lower jaw is too far forward or whether your face is too elongated. The photos can show when there's a skeletal issue such as a severe overjet, which is an upper jaw that's too far forward, or an underbite, which is a lower jaw that's too far forward. Problems such as these may require more than simply moving teeth within the bone, they may require jaw surgery or other, more complex procedures in the treatment plan.

Cephalometric radiographs (x-rays) in 2-D and/or 3-D imaging show measurements of the head and can show how the various parts of your face and teeth relate to each other. Cone beam computed tomography (CBCT) also delivers a

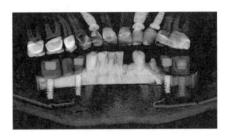

3-D image of the head and neck. These are extremely sophisticated technologies that show teeth and bone struc-tures, even under the gums.

These technologies may also reveal when a patient has a breathing problem, potentially as a result of developmental issues or allergic reactions. When there's a breathing problem, treatment is likely going to include orthodontics and possibly surgery. The goal at that point is to save the patient's life, because *breathing is the only option.*

Work with the lab or orthodontist. Once there's an accurate picture of any issues you are experiencing, then the digital files are used to communicate and design and fine tune a plan according to the dentist's prescription. Lab techs set up treatment in a virtual setting, while the dentist and/or orthodontist determines the function and aesthetic outcome.

Treatment files are passed back and forth, sometimes several times, before the final braces or aligners are approved by the dentist and then created at the lab. If the treatment appears to be very complex, we always collaborate with a specialist to create the most ideal result.

Address health issues. Part of pre-treatment involves looking at other problems in your mouth, including tooth decay or gum disease. The goal is to remove any bacteria from teeth and gums so that everything is healthy while the braces or clear aligners are doing their work.

In some cases, however, a tooth may have a temporary, protective treatment done until all your teeth are aligned. For instance, if a tooth needs extensive strengthening internally due to decay, a filling or temporary crown may be placed until the tooth has been moved to its proper position. At that point, a permanent crown will be placed. Determining whether a tooth is strong enough to withstand orthodontics, or whether it needs to be treated first, is part of preparation for treatment.

Keeping Your Mouth Healthy

During the straightening process, inflammation and decay must be kept at bay so that your teeth will have healthy gums and bone in which to move. Daily flossing—which can be a challenge with braces—and regular cleanings by a hygienist can help teeth and gums stay in good condition.

A re-mineralizing toothpaste can also help keep teeth avoid decalcification or cavities and keep enamel stain-free. It's also important to manage what's known as the "biofilm" in your mouth. The biofilm is the sludge of bacteria that permeates the body—including the mouth.

TIPS FOR A HEALTHY MOUTH DURING STRAIGHTENING

· Floss daily

· Get regular cleanings by a hygienist

· Use a re-mineralizing toothpaste

· Manage your biofilm

In spite of all the fluoride that is put into city drinking water, people still get cavities these days. That's because the acidity in your mouth becomes a magnet to pull calcium and phosphate outside the tooth. When that happens, the tooth starts to break down; it starts to get softer, usually on the inside. But re-mineralizing can help reverse some of the damage that's just getting started. When a patient is going through orthodontics, "remineralization" can help reverse some of the damage from poor brushing—brushing that leaves debris. That debris can promote more acid in the mouth, and lead to damage around the brackets or in between the teeth.

To manage the health of the mouth, I use products from CariFree, a company that produces pH-elevated products that are scientifically proven to prevent cavities because they change the chemical balance of the mouth. The company has invested in researching its products, and they are extremely effective.

Keeping Teeth Straight

Once your teeth are straightened, then the goal is to keep them aligned by ensuring that the bone tightens up around them. Retainers can keep teeth in place for the long term when worn correctly.

Most of the time, retainers these days are clear trays, very much like clear aligner treatment. These retainers are made at an orthodontic lab from a digital scan of the teeth after straightening. Or, in some practices, retainers are printed in-house on a 3-D printer.

Retainers should be worn full time for about three months in order to stabilize the teeth.

However, once your teeth are straightened, your bite may still need to be balanced. To make those adjustments, I use technology known as a Kois Deprogrammer, a removable appliance that relaxes the muscles and evaluates the bite, muscles, and the jaw joint. The deprogrammer allows jaw muscles to relax and settle into the ideal position as they relate to the temporomandibular joint (TMJ). The TMJs are the joints on either side of your face that connect your jawbone to your skull. The deprogrammer appliance is worn daily for at least one to two weeks for at least four to five hours. Then, using a technique called **bite equilibration**, special papers are inserted in between your teeth to measure contact points and any areas of friction that might cause teeth or veneers to chip or gums to recede and become inflamed. Minimal corrections are then made with a polishing instrument to preserve as much tooth structure as possible. Another benefit of equilibration is that it can reduce teeth sensitivity, as well as head and neck pain because it helps to calm muscle and nerve pathways.

Once the bite is balanced, then esthetic planning can begin. That may include whitening, contouring your teeth and/or gums, bonding some teeth, or applying veneers. It all comes down to individual needs and wants.

How Long Does It All Take?

The timeline for treatments is customized to each patient's needs, wants, and other factors. For instance, a person's health and other factors, such as how quickly some of their teeth will move, can be determining factors in how long their treatment takes.

Compliance is also a factor: One of the drawbacks of the aligner system is that it's up to the patient to wear their aligners for twenty-two hours a day. They should only be removed for eating, brushing, and flossing.

Today, **artificial intelligence** (AI) is helping eliminate some of the problems with compliance. Many aligner systems on the market have come out with some extremely advanced technology called "Dental Monitoring." The technology involves the patient using a retractor along with an app on their phone to take photos and videos of their mouth that are automatically sent to the dentist or orthodontist providing treatment. Those videos help the dentist stay on top of the patient's treatment. The data collected by the videos lets the dentist know whether it's time to see the patient for a repair or to tweak the treatment and it can send the patient a reminder to get back on track with their treatment or even give them a "pat on the back" for doing a good job following the treatment plan and start with the next aligner. Eventually, AI will be used for other things in dentistry to better serve you and your health, as well as appearance needs. Stay tuned at https://www.DrHughFlax.com.

Whatever the method used, the best way to straighten teeth is to follow the instructions given by your dental provider regarding office visits, changing the trays as prescribed, and keeping your recommended dental cleanings.

David's Smile—A Powerful Image

David followed the instructions for his treatment and ended up with a smile befitting his place behind the wheel of some of the world's most powerful and prestigious cars.

Putting your teeth into teeth in the right places not only improves your appearance, it also decreases the chances of further wear and tear on your teeth. Naturally, people often want to fix previous chips and wear or close spaces with bonding or contouring the enamel. The next chapter contains some helpful insights on these procedures.

SMILE ON!

What can you do now to further explore straightening your teeth?

- See an accredited cosmetic dentist with training in functional dentistry to properly evaluate your bite and determine whether you need an orthodontic solution. The Kois Center, The Pankey Institute, The Dawson Academy, and Spear Education offer training in functional dentistry.

- If your situation is complex, see a well-respected orthodontist to be evaluated and collaborate with a cosmetic dentist. That can make all the difference in your treatment outcomes.

- Avoid solutions that aren't supervised by a qualified dentist, such as do-it-yourself online or mail-order clubs—like the ones that you see on television.

CHAPTER 4

BONDING AND CONTOURING— A SIMPLE SOLUTION

Anna was in her senior year in college and looking forward to going to grad school in Fort Lauderdale when she fell down and traumatized her two front teeth. Using the CBCT x-ray, I was able to three dimensionally determine the amount of damage, which was quite extensive. Her teeth were chipped and pushed back up into the bone in her mouth, challenges that would require an orchestrated team of multiple specialists to help repair correctly and in a timely manner.

I sent her to an oral surgeon to repair the bone in order to stabilize her teeth. After the bone had healed, she went to an orthodontist to move her teeth back into place. Then she also went to an endodontist to have root canal treatments on both traumatized teeth. We knew that there was a chance that she could have even more problems with those teeth in the future as a result of biological changes, such as bone loss that weakened the support around the teeth. That could mean the need for implants if things started to breakdown.

After all the other treatments were completed and her teeth were stabilized (thankfully, before graduation), it was time to repair the damage with cosmetic dentistry. Since her teeth were intact, yet there was a chance that she could have trouble in the future with those teeth, then the best solution for Anna was not crowns, but bonding. Crowns would have required removing a lot of the tooth structure, while bonding was a conservative option to make her look whole and beautiful again without fully committing to such a dramatic, permanent, and costly solution as crowns.

In short, I was buying time. At such a young age, it can be a big spend for parents to help their child restore her smile. So, bonding gave Anna and her parents some breathing room. Later, if Anna's teeth need upgrading, then ideally, she will have the resources to take care of the treatment out of her own pocket. Footing the bill later in life will let her appreciate the value of her investment even more.

"I can't even begin to express how great my experience has been being a patient of Dr. Flax and his team members. After my mouth injury, I was panicking thinking that my teeth would never look normal again. Dr. Flax was able to squeeze me into his busy schedule soon after my injury and connect me to other healthcare professionals who would take care of my mouth as well. Not only were Dr. Flax and his team members able to repair my damaged teeth, but they were able to make them look even better than they did prior to my injury. Thank you to Dr. Flax and his team members! I will be forever grateful!"

—Anna

See Anna's progress in the before and after photo section.

Bonding and Contouring—The Basics

When it comes to determining treatment for a patient, we look at their overall, long-term goals. They might ask about having one tooth treated, but by talking with them and listening, we may find that they are unhappy with other teeth as well. It's not about selling teeth, I just want to "shepherd patients to the promised land"—what is the overall goal versus the immediate want? Yes, we can fix one broken front tooth, but we have a lot of technologies today that can deliver a better smile than they ever imagined. At the same time, I don't want to just put a menu of options before a patient and ask them to choose—I want to help them understand that they have options, what those options are, and what the consequences of their choices might be.

Bonding and contouring are two cosmetic dentistry procedures that can deliver big results with minimal changes and cost.

Bonding is an additive process that beautifies and strengthens tooth structure. Your teeth have natural porosities in the outer enamel and inner dentin. Cleaning these tubules and impregnating them with resin liquids called **bonding agents** allows them to become sticky enough to hold tooth-colored materials of varying strengths and colors. The goal of bonding is to replace lost or missing tooth structure so, using different colors and densities of material, bonding rebuilds the shapes, contours, shades, and stratification of the tooth to make it look as natural as possible.

THREE INDICATIONS FOR BONDING

· Worn or chipped teeth

· Small spaces between teeth—ideally the space is no more than three millimeters in diameter

· Areas of decay in the front or back of the mouth

Bonding replaces enamel that has been worn away due to factors such as damage or aging. Cases that are ideal for bonding are those where there is a bit of enamel or exterior of the tooth worn away, but not so much that the inner layer of the tooth, the dentin, is exposed. When a lot of enamel is worn away and the dentin is exposed, then porcelain veneers or crowns may be a better option. I'll talk more about veneers in the next chapter.

When done right, bonding can last a long time; it's reasonable for bonding to last up to eight to ten years—occasionally longer. But that means addressing a number of other factors. For instance, if the bite is off, bonding is more prone to chipping or being worn down. In addition, if there are bone issues or problems with the gums, the teeth can shift. But if all those risk factors are addressed first, then the teeth can be prepared properly, the bonding applied, and finally everything polished to create a beautiful, long-lasting smile.

Too often, bonding gets a bad rap because the patient has other problems that are not addressed first, so they have a shaky foundation to start with. "Form follows function," so treatment should begin by managing the risk factors, such as a good bite and healthy teeth, bone, and gums.

Contouring is a reductive procedure. It involves reshaping tooth structure to very conservatively smooth or improve the esthetic appearance or functional bite forces for better long-term results. Since it is a reductive process that involves taking away some of the tooth structure, it is kept to a minimum to avoid compromising the outer, white enamel. If too much contouring is needed, orthodontics may be a better lifelong option.

Depending on the strategy, contouring may involve shortening a tooth, shaping the corners (the embrasures) to have a softer appearance, trimming up unevenness—just giving back some youthfulness to the teeth.

Planning the design of the smile and esthetic begins by making a digital or solid model of the teeth, as well as photos and any necessary x-rays, to study where to "nip and tuck" to create the illusion or the appearance that the patient desires.

After planning the design of a smile that matches esthetic and durability goals, the teeth are conservatively contoured and polished to more ideal shapes or positioned. Then the bonding is added to augment colors, repair chips, close spaces, etc. so that teeth appear and feel better. This can take from one to three visits, depending on a patient's needs.

Bonding—A Good Choice for Some, Not for Others

There are a number of reasons to choose bonding as an option for a beautiful smile.

With a teen, who is still growing. Since it is a conservative option, bonding is a good choice for teens getting ready to graduate high school. Teens' bodies are still changing, and they often are not mature enough to take responsibility for their teeth. So, veneers are not a good choice when bonding will do.

As a transition before veneers. When a patient is not quite ready for veneers—maybe they still have enough tooth to salvage—then bonding can be better choice. Bonding can also buy more time for someone that doesn't quite have the budget for veneers or crowns.

When teeth are chipped but structure remains. Bonding is better if there is at least two-thirds of the tooth remaining. It is usually a better solution for a chipped tooth versus cutting it down for a veneer or crown, and then hoping the lab can match up the adjacent teeth. Bonding is what I'd choose for my child should they have a chipped tooth that needs repair. Teeth that are badly broken down or that have had a root canal may instead need a porcelain treatment, such as a crown.

With a challenging need to match tooth color, texture, or shape. The "holy grail of cosmetic dentistry" is to try to match up a piece of porcelain to one tooth—that's extremely difficult to do, especially in the front of the mouth. Bonding allows for colors to be layered to come up with an attractive result, one that makes the patient feel good again.

At the same time, bonding may not last forever. Whether to use it depends on the condition of the tooth. It worked for Anna, in part because several dental professionals were able to work together to save her teeth. But if there has been chipping and stress on the teeth for many years, so much that the teeth have fractured or there is chronic microtrauma, then other procedures may need to be considered.

With non-staining diets. Smoking, red wine, coffee, and other staining agents are less than ideal with bonding. That's because the material can stain, but it cannot be whitened. So, consuming red wine or coffee, or smoking, can cause unattractive and irreversible discolorations.

When the bite is in good shape. Bruxers—people who clench and grind their teeth—are not good candidates for bonding. That's why we try to correct bite issues early, before we place any bonding. When bonding is done on someone that has bruxing issues, it will be a short-term treatment.

When budget is a factor. Bonding is a more economical solution for repair of teeth that are worn or chipped. Porcelain procedures such as veneers or crowns can cost three times as much as bonding due to the time involved and the costs of using the lab that fabricates the materials. However, when a person is not a good candidate for bonding, then the more ideal solution could be porcelain veneers. I'll talk more about these in the next chapter.

Affordable Fixes for Anna

For Anna, bonding and contouring were the best solutions for giving back her smile after it was traumatized from a fall. These treatments were affordable fixes after orthodontics and endodontic procedures repaired damage to her front teeth. Later, when she has more resources of her own and as the treatment ages, she may want to pursue more permanent solutions.

For patients with busy lives, porcelain veneers may be a better option since the treatment can be even longer lasting than bonding—I have one patient who has been in veneers since 1989. Veneers offer more bang for the dollar than bonding, making them potentially a better investment for patients who want a long-term, beautiful smile.

SMILE ON!

What can you do now to further explore bonding for your teeth?

- Visit www.AACD.com to find an accredited cosmetic dentist to evaluate and help you plan a realistic treatment.

- Make sure your teeth and gums are healthy and strong (see chapter 9).

- Look for photos of actual patients and read their testimonials about their bonding experience.

CHAPTER 5

VENEERS CAN HELP YOU LOOK AND FEEL YOUNGER

Michelle first came to see me because she wanted to learn more about laser treatment for her children. While we were talking about treatment for them, she noticed the photos of patients that had been treated that we have hanging around the office. Seeing their outcomes, she asked if I would talk with her about her own smile.

She was already a very attractive woman, but when she smiled, she had teeth that were angled and chipped. She didn't have a "whole smile," and it had bothered her for many years. Even though her friends would tell her she looked fine, she knew her teeth were taking away from her smile. She consulted with several dentists, but was told that the only way to align her teeth was jaw surgery. "That's how we'll move your teeth, so you won't have to wear braces," they all told her.

Since she had a corporate job, and she felt that there had to be a less-aggressive option; she wanted to see what I might be able to do.

Using veneers on her ten upper teeth, we were able to change the angles and display of the teeth to create the illusion that they were straight, while also building volume so that she had a nice, full smile. We didn't have to remove a lot of tooth structure, and it only required some mild contouring of her gums to give her a gorgeous smile. We did it all without any major surgery or tooth loss, for which she was extremely grateful.

Her finished smile was so outstanding that her case is featured quite often in literature on veneers, and she was even on the cover of the *Journal of Cosmetic Dentistry*.

See Michelle's progress in the before and after photo section.

A New Smile—A New You

Just as the body changes over time, so do teeth. But most people don't realize the changes that occur—they just look in the mirror one day and realize that their teeth are worn, chipped, discolored, and dull.

Veneers are custom-made, tooth-colored shell coverings. They are uniform shapes and colored based on where they are located in the mouth, so they create a very pleasing, symmetrical smile. They are made of porcelain, which is very durable and natural-looking—it mimics your tooth structure. When bonded to your teeth, veneers change the appearance of your whole smile.

Veneers offer a conservative way to preserve the natural functional anatomy and strength of a tooth. They reinvigorate the exterior of the tooth, making it stronger, more luminous, and more youthful again.

Veneers fit tightly to the tooth structure, replacing enamel that has become worn and damaged. They can add length and strength to a tooth while masking its defects. They can even be crafted to close gaps in teeth. And they resist discoloration from wine, cigarettes, coffee, and other staining agents.

When done correctly, veneers can easily last twenty to twenty-five years. As I mentioned earlier, I have one patient whose veneers have been intact for more than thirty years.

The actual process of treating with veneers is multilayered. It's almost like having somebody design and customize a Tesla or a Corvette just for you.

As Dr. Pascal Magne explains in his dental textbook, *Bonded Porcelain Restorations in the Anterior Dentition: A Biomimetic Approach*, the front teeth are thicker on the backside. This part of the tooth anatomy, known as the **cingulum**, keeps the front teeth from flexing and breaking. When the cingulum is removed, it dramatically weakens the teeth, making them more prone to cracking. When removing any cingulum from a crown, it is critical that a reinforcing base of 2 mm of vertical and horizontal natural tooth structure (a ferrule effect) remains to prevent any changes.[17]

The goal, then, when rejuvenating front teeth, is to save as much of the cingulum as possible. Veneers allow for the cingulum to be retained, preserving vital tooth structure, whereas crowns require more tooth structure to be removed, which can weaken the tooth in the long run. That's one of the distinct advantages of having a veneer versus a crown—less enamel is removed.

---

17   Pascal Magne and Urs Belser, *Bonded Porcelain Restorations in the Anterior Dentition: A Biomimetic Approach* (Batavia, Illinois: Quintessence Publishing Co. Inc., 2002), 23–53.

Tooth enamel may be two or three millimeters thick. During the veneer preparation process, oftentimes six- to eight-tenths of a millimeter of the enamel may be removed to make room for the very thin wafer of porcelain veneer. That veneer is designed to fit on the tooth almost like a contact lens fits on the eye. When fitted to the existing tooth, which is polished as part of the preparation process, the veneer creates a tight seal that can protect the tooth because the porcelain is so durable—it will not crack and does not stain.

In some cases, we do minimal or no prep for veneers. That typically involves ultra-thin veneers, known by brand names such as Lumineers or DURAthins. These are not ideal for all cases. They are quite conservative, and often best done to build volume or close spaces to avoid making the tooth look a little boxy or square—it's more difficult to take advantage of shapes and contours of existing teeth to create a more natural-looking smile.

In fact, the look of veneers often comes down to the dentist's relationship with their lab tech. Veneers are crafted at the lab based on the details of the treatment that the dentist shares after examining the patient. Today's digital technologies allow for much better collaboration between dentist and lab tech, making the back-and-forth exchange of information when tailoring veneers quick and easy. I've had the same lab tech—a master ceramist—for two decades, and we've collaboratively taught each other a few things over the years.

Getting Veneers

A veneer procedure is really about implementing the architectural and esthetic game plan that is created in collaboration with the patient. The process starts by talking about the image you're trying to project, what you dream for your ideal smile. Do you want to repair some damage? Do you want a more uniform look? Do you want to turn back the clock? Sometimes we will do Digital Smile Design and a mockup with video to verify we are on the same page. Then, we create a model of your teeth using either digital or solid modeling. Part of this planning stage involves understanding both how the smile will look and how it will function. Each patient's smile must not only be beautiful and believable, but it also must last a long time.

Every veneer treatment comes with a "test drive." By first applying prototypes, or temporary veneers, you're able to see how your new smile looks and how it feels to chew and speak. When the temporaries are in place, potential problems are identified. Do the teeth look real? Does the bite and speech feel comfortable? Are the veneers in danger of chipping? If any of these potential problems exist, then they must be resolved before moving forward. Prototypes create a safety net for patients so that they can get long-term joy and endurance out of their smile. It's almost a religious commitment to get the engineering and the prototypes just right before having the laboratory move forward with making the final porcelain.

Using prototypes also gives you an idea of how other people will react to your new smile. The goal is to have people see a new-and-improved you, but without knowing exactly what was done. A real win is when a friend says, "You look happier and more relaxed. I don't know why, but you look fantastic!"

That's the secret to great cosmetic dentistry: Unless your smile was pretty severely degraded beforehand, your new smile shouldn't be so dazzling that it's apparent you had it made over. In other words, you should enter the room before your smile does, not the other way around.

Veneers are ideal for teeth that are beyond the point of being rejuvenated with bonding. However, if too much of the tooth structure is missing or unstable, then veneers are likely not an option. When more than half of the enamel is gone, then a crown may be the best solution. At that point, however, we investigate why the enamel is gone—is it from friction? Misaligned teeth? Is it chemical changes caused by certain drinks? Is there a health issue such as bulimia or gastric reflux?

The Materials

As I've mentioned, while the veneers themselves cover discolorations, the porcelain material they are made of is impervious to stains. That's unlike natural tooth structure, which has porosities that pick-up stains from smoking and drinking wine, coffee, and other staining agents. For that reason, some of our patients like to have the bottom teeth veneered as well—with veneers top and bottom, you can eat berries and tomato sauce and drink coffee and wine without worrying about staining. Whether you're in Napa or at the Waffle House, your smile will always look great!

There are different types of porcelain used for restorative treatments, such as veneers.

The classic porcelain is **feldspathic**, but more modern types of porcelain include **zirconia**, **pressed ceramic**, and **lithium disilicate**. A commonly used pressed ceramic is a product known as IPS Empress, and commonly used lithium disilicate products include IPS e.max or LiSi Press. The materials keep evolving, and they've improved over the years. So, I now have more choices for added durability and function than previously available.

The type of porcelain used depends on the tooth structure being replaced, basically where the tooth is located in the mouth and what surfaces show in the smile. For instance, veneers made from feldspathic porcelain have optical characteristics that closely match the beauty and warmth of natural teeth, so that material may be used for outside surfaces of the front teeth. Yet its weaker strength is less favorable in high-stress areas of the mouth. With front teeth that are worn or chipped, the stronger lithium disilicate may be a better choice because veneers made of this material can add to the length of the affected teeth while holding up to the forces.

Zirconia, meanwhile, is often the choice for a crown in the back of the mouth, where the teeth need to be stronger. Although it has a nice luster, it is not as esthetically pleasing as lithium disilicate or feldspathic. In addition, zirconia requires more tooth reduction—a millimeter and a half to two millimeters—which is more than necessary for a conservative veneer. Lastly, sometimes lithium disilicate is used when doing an inlay or onlay, a conservative technique that refurbishes a back tooth but doesn't require a crown.

Why does all this technical stuff about porcelain matter? Because it's important to use the right strength of material to create the longest lasting, most beautiful smile you can have.

How Many Veneers Are Right for You?

When you smile, you tend to display more of your upper teeth. When talking, more of your lower teeth show. But the brain detects when there's a difference—if you're talking to someone who is also smiling, it can be very distracting when their upper and lower teeth don't match. In fact, when veneers aren't done optimally, it can create a distracting, rather than attractive, smile. Perhaps you've seen a celebrity with gleaming white, youthful-looking teeth in the front but stained and older-looking teeth on the sides of their smile? That's because they only had a minimal number of teeth rejuvenated in the front, which can leave all the stained and darker teeth showing on the sides of the mouth. That can even make it appear that some back teeth are missing. YIKES.

Too often, veneers are only applied to the front six teeth, as many of us were taught in dental school in the 1980s.

But I look at the mouth as being like a "Broadway play," an analogy I use courtesy of my colleague, Dr. Larry Rosenthal, "a dentist to the stars." Imagine that the teeth are the actors on the stage, and all the front teeth (especially the front two) are the stars of the show. Still, you can't ignore the supporting actors—the teeth on the sides of the mouth. Nor can you ignore the scenery (the gums) or the curtains (the lips).

So if you have veneers only on the six upper front teeth, then your lower front teeth and all the supporting actors can be less youthful-looking. And while whitening can brighten teeth that do not have veneers, it may be temporary solution. Plus, it may be impossible to whiten stained teeth to match the color and shine of the veneers. That's why the best smile comes from having veneers applied to the teeth that you display in your smile—usually eight to ten teeth in the front, and potentially the lower teeth.

Michelle's Model Smile

Michelle's treatment was so amazing that it made her a star and landed her on the cover of a magazine. With veneers—instead of far more aggressive jaw surgery—she was able to get the smile she had longed for.

Again, the teeth may be the stars and the supporting actors of the show, but there are other players on the stage that must also get attention when rejuvenating a smile. **Gum reshaping**, also referred to as **gum contouring** or a **gum lift**, can create more symmetry in your smile and make your stars shine brighter.

SMILE ON!

What can you do right now if you want to look and feel younger through veneers?

- Research the best accredited cosmetic dentist in your area.

- Ask to see photos of actual patient cases.

- Find out who the dentist uses as a lab for their veneer cases.

CHAPTER 6

A GUM LIFT—
A GORGEOUS WAY TO
CREATE SMILE SYMMETRY

After seeing the photos of her son's wedding, Hazel realized that she never smiled at all. It was upsetting to know that, at such a memorable event, the photos to commemorate it would never reflect the happiness she felt inside. But that's what it took to motivate Hazel to do something about her sixty-two-year-old smile.

An evaluation of her smile revealed that she would need multi-disciplinary care—orthodontics and a gum lift—before her veneers and crowns. But after I presented the treatment options to her, she decided to forgo having anything done. At her age, she said, she had already lived with a lifetime of problems, so she felt the investment wasn't worth it.

To motivate her and give her some hope, I asked whether she'd like to see a 3-D blueprint of her new smile that would let her see the possibilities. When she saw what her smile could be, she said, "Doc, let's do it." As a very down-to-earth person, she also added, perhaps as an extra incentive to me, "If you do a good job, I'll pray for you. If you do a bad job, I'm going to pray against you."

Step by step, we really created a miracle in her mouth. With orthodontics, we corrected a sizable gap in her teeth. And then by recontouring her gums, we were able to give her a smile that was far more symmetrical—a smile she happily showed wherever she went.

Perhaps what's most significant about Hazel's story is that, a few months after her treatments were finished, she came back to see us and I didn't even recognize her. She had changed her hairstyle, lost about thirty pounds by exercising, was in much better shape physically, and she was no longer wearing glasses. The transformation was incredible—her cosmetic dentistry results had triggered a landslide of self-improvement.

See Hazel's progress in the before and after photo section.

Gum Lifts—Art and Biology

As I mentioned earlier, I view the mouth as being like a Broadway play. While the teeth are the actors on that stage, the gums are the scenery—an important part of the overall production. Gums that are asymmetrical, bulky in one area, short or long on a tooth here or there, or leaving teeth without a pleasing frame can disrupt the eye of the viewer—it can be distracting to talk with someone when their gums are unbalanced or unhealthy. Pink, healthy, and symmetrical gums can make a big difference in a smile.

A gum lift can revitalize the gums and make the gumline far more pleasing. It involves reshaping gum tissue and/or bone to improve smile esthetics. Gum lifts can create the illusion of straightness in the smile and even up the symmetry around the teeth to provide more natural architecture that "frames" the teeth better to dramatically enhance the smile.

As you can imagine, there is an art to creating the ideal gumline.

Creating a natural-looking smile means following the laws of nature. Those laws dictate that the gums have symmetry, balance, and a geometric progression from the front to the back of the mouth.[18] To achieve harmony with the gums during contouring, specific ratios and angles should be followed. For instance, the two upper front teeth, known as the central incisors, should have a ratio of 75 to 80 percent width to length to avoid looking too long or too square.[19]

"Embrasures" are the V-shaped areas at the edges and gumlines where the teeth come together. These create angles that should go from acute in the front of the mouth to obtuse at the back. These elements will create a pleasing and natural scallop effect—the tissue heights of the central incisors will match that of the canines (the upper teeth third from center on either side) while the gumline of the lateral incisors (the teeth on either side of the central incisors) is just slightly shorter.

After determining the smile design with computer imaging and digital smile design, the gums (and potentially the bone) are conservatively reshaped to remove excess or uneven gum tissue, a procedure known as a "closed flap." The procedure is often done using a diode or erbium laser to "nip and tuck" in different places to create symmetry. Many dentists use a lower-powered diode laser for this procedure, which targets only the gum tissue. But an erbium laser has at least more than twice the power of the diode, which allows for issues with the gum *and* the bone to be addressed—often in one visit.

---

18   Claude Rufenacht, *Fundamentals of Esthetics* (Batavia, Illinois: Quintessence Publishing Co. Inc., 1990).

19   G. J. Chiche and A. Pinault, *Esthetics of Anterior Fixed Prosthodontics* (Batavia, Illinois: Quintessence Publishing Co. Inc., 1994).

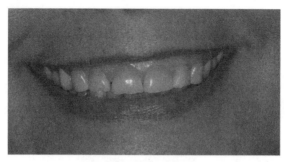

BEFORE

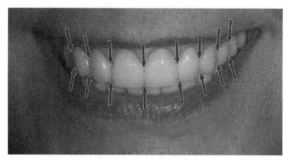

AFTER

USING A LASER AND SMILE DESIGN PRINCIPLES
ALLOWED US TO IMPROVE THE ESTHETIC
PROPORTIONS AND EMBRASURES
(INDICATED BY ARROWS IN THE "AFTER" IMAGE)
TO ENHANCE OUR PATIENT'S SMILE.

When more changes are needed for the teeth and gums, then **open-flap** surgery may be required. By "opening" the gum tissue, more dramatic modifications can be made, such as correcting recession by adding volume to the tissues or repairing tooth and bone structure for better health and esthetics. While less-complex issues can be addressed with the **closed-flap** procedure, very complicated problems are referred to a periodontist. That can mean delaying other cosmetic dentistry because of the logistics of using multiple providers and the time involved in healing from the more intensive surgery. If we recommend this, it is worth the small inconvenience for enjoying the long-term benefit.

Now, let's look at the science of a gum lift.

When the teeth and gums are healthy, there is a biologic width between the gum and the bone. In 85 to 90 percent of patients, that depth of the **pocket**, as it is known, from edge of the gums to the crest of the bone is three millimeters, and the gum/bone thickness is more resistant to recession when it is thinner.[20] Oftentimes, a dental laser can be used to reduce excess gum tissue and then smooth the recontoured gums. Sometimes, to achieve the proper biologic width with gum sculpting, as previously mentioned, the bone must be moved with either a closed-flap procedure (performed with a laser or a small metal instrument called a chisel), or with an open-flap surgery. Closed-flap procedures can be performed during veneer treatment, allowing smiles to be completed faster and with predictable results. That is something that has to be planned for when you and your cosmetic team meet.

While there are guidelines to follow when contouring, each patient's gumline is unique. The goal with the finished smile is to have symmetry at the midline but some asymmetry along the sides, creating a pleasing blend of the ideal smile with natural irregularities—that's what makes a smile look natural and realistic, as opposed to looking like a row of dentures made from a template.

The art of contouring is a little like driving a car. There are rules of the road, but there are also times where instinctual decisions must

---

20   John Kois, "Altering Gingival Levels: The Restorative Connection, Part I: Biologic Variables," *Journal of Esthetic and Restorative Dentistry* 6, no. 1 (July 2007): 3–7, https://doi.org/10.1111/j.1708-8240.1994.tb00825.x.

be made that are in the best interest of the occupants of the car—or, in the case of gum contouring, the patient. That's something that the dentist learns over time by working with thousands of patients and developing a level of mastery by putting in tens of thousands of hours performing gum lifts. Because there are limits to artistry when working with the biology of the mouth, and fighting against the laws of nature is a losing battle—that's why it's important to know the parameters and to have the instincts and experience to know what works.

Risks? Yes, Some

With any dental procedure, there is a risk of infection. Following a gum lift, patients must participate in their care.

To help with rapid and successful healing, patients are given detailed care information that includes verbal and written instructions to follow. Caring for the gums after treatment includes careful flossing and using an aloe and antibacterial gel to help with healing. We also provide an instrument that we call a **rubber tip** for patients to use in massaging their gum tissues to firm everything up after surgery.

The beauty of using laser is that it provides a precise cut that instantly reshapes the tissue, which minimizes bleeding and leaves no necrosis or injured tissue as in older techniques like "electrosurgery." The result is quicker healing time and better overall results.

Still, gum contouring can be somewhat complex. So, to stay within biologic parameters, adjustments commonly require two or more visits. The first visit typically involves the initial closed-flap technique. Then, when veneer treatment starts, additional gum shaping or bone adjustment may be needed to aid in healing. There is a lot of checking back and forth to ensure that everything is turning out as expected because biology is involved, so sometimes the target shifts a little. That's the body adapting to changes and is one reason why patient participation is so important to ensure a successful outcome.

Most patients report minimal discomfort with gum lifting procedures. In fact, we commonly hear patients say, "I can't believe it was that easy."

Turning Back the Clock for Hazel

For Hazel and others like her, a gum lift can turn back the clock and truly give them something to smile about. All it takes is a little homework to find a qualified, quality cosmetic dentist or periodontist to perform the procedure, because gum lifts by themselves can be very predictable.

But since the mouth also involves the forces of the teeth fitting together, you need a healthy bite to keep a gum lift stable over the long haul. In the next chapter, I'll talk about what makes a good bite, and treatments to help correct your bite and keep it stable.

SMILE ON!

What are some easy first steps for you to begin transforming your smile?

- Take care of your gums to keep them healthy.

- Replace any dental issues that are working against you having healthy gums such as areas of decay or bulky, ill-fitting fillings, or crowns.

- Find out the level of expertise and technology that your treating dentist has for performing gum lifts. Ask to see pictures of previous, actual patients and credentials of training, certification, or teaching.

CHAPTER 7

HOW TO MAKE YOUR SMILE LAST LONGER AND CHEW COMFORTABLY

J ackie struggled with pain in her jaw muscles for many years. When she first came to see me and we evaluated her issues, we realized that the problem was her bite, and that improving the bite was going to require two steps. The first step was to align her teeth to resolve both health and esthetic issues and the second was to balance her bite so that the peaks and valleys of her teeth fit together.

We treated her with Invisalign for nine months. After that, she wore her retainers for three months to allow her teeth to tighten up. Then we adjusted her bite using the Kois Deprogrammer. Afterward, Jackie was able to live pain-free.

"After years of struggling with jaw pain and difficulty chewing, I finally found Dr. Flax. He was extremely thorough in his examination and took many pictures of my teeth from every angle in addition to creating molds. He explained to me that my issues seemed to stem not only from the fact that my bite was off but also that I clench my jaw constantly. Not a single one of the many

dentists I had seen over the years had even suggested to me that this could be the problem and the reason for my pain. None had ever taken the time or effort that Dr. Flax did to find the source of my chronic discomfort. … Dr. Flax and his staff ensured I had the results I wanted and all my teeth were where they should be. … I trusted his ability and his judgement. When he was done, I could not believe I could bite down properly for the first time since I can remember. He totally 'blew my mind!'

"Dr. Flax and all of his staff are absolutely amazing people. I'm very happy that after all these years I finally found a dental practice that truly cares!"

—*Jackie*

What Causes a Bad Bite?

According to Dr. Peter Dawson, one of the world's leading experts on creating a balanced bite:

> For the average patient, dentistry is all about teeth, so they spend an inordinate amount of time brushing, flossing, and rinsing—which is obviously a terrific first step toward maintaining healthy teeth. However, what the average patient is not aware of is that brushing, flossing, and rinsing are just a part of the process for maintaining healthy teeth. In reality, each and every component of the masticatory system, which consists of the anterior teeth, posterior teeth, muscles, and temporomandibular joints (TMJs), must also be maintained in good health. That's because each component of the masticatory system must function together. If any part of the system does not function properly, it will have a profound ripple effect on the

remaining parts of the system, including muscle pain, worn teeth, headaches, and countless other problems.[21]

A bad bite (or **malocclusion**) is one where the upper and lower teeth don't come together smoothly and comfortably free of excessive muscle tension without overloading the anatomy and strength of the teeth, gums, bone, jaw joints, and nerves.

A bad bite can be caused by any number of factors. Here are some of the primary reasons we see bad bites:

External factors, such as how you process events in your life. Maybe you're overstimulated by things such as social media or the news. Whatever the external factor is, it may be causing you to clench or grind your teeth.

Problems sleeping can cause bite problems. If a person has trouble breathing when they sleep, it can be caused by a collapsing airway. To keep the airway open, teeth naturally clench. Since "breathing is not an option," you must be able to breathe whether awake or asleep. When a patient tells me that they don't feel energized when they wake up or they wake every morning with a sore jaw, then I know they are likely having sleep and breathing problems. We used to think it was because of external stress, but there's an internal stress of not being able to breathe.

Bad habits, such as chewing on your nails or biting a pencil.

Social habits like taking illegal drugs or having an eating disorder like bulimia can wreak havoc on the teeth and ruin an otherwise good bite.

---

21   Peter E. Dawson, "Dawson Quicknotes," The Dawson Academy, accessed March 20, 2019, https://thedawsonacademy.typepad.com/quicknotes/2008/12/clinical-assisting-for-occlusal-equilibration.html.

Biologic problems include disorders of the stomach, such as gastric reflux or GERD, and low pH in the mouth. These can lead to a bad bite.

Genetics is another factor behind a bad bite. There's a physiological level of adaptation that human automatically go through when born. From the moment a baby emerges from the womb, their body begins adapting to the environment. The way a jaw develops and/or the alignment of teeth affects the way they interact with each other.

At any given point in time, the body is making micro-decisions and using feedback mechanisms for survival. Sometimes, that can impact the teeth in a negative way. That's why dentists try to help people adapt to the world better—because their bodies are doing that all the time.

Friction—Small Movements Create Big Problems

Teeth can become loose because of bone loss, but they also loosen because of friction. Friction is a small issue that can lead to big problems. When you bite your teeth together and chew, can you feel your teeth moving? That's friction, a type of micromovement in the mouth that is known as **fremitus.** Even though it's slight, if not corrected, it can have devastating consequences. It can cause significant wear and tear and even create bite problems. If you're having trouble chewing tough foods, like bagels or steak, it might be caused by jaw muscles not working together or teeth that do not fit together well—and that can cause friction. Most friction is so subtle that it goes unnoticed.

Try this test: Take your forefinger and touch your two front teeth or any of your teeth about halfway back in your mouth. Now clench and grind your teeth just a little. Do you feel even a slight movement of the tooth you are touching? That's friction.

It can be a little scary to realize there is movement in your teeth. It's scary for me, too, especially when I'm about to begin treatment and then find that there is micromovement in one or more teeth. When friction is found, it is corrected before moving forward.

SIGNS OF A BAD BITE

Signs in the mouth can indicate when there is an issue with the bite. These signs can also cause bite issues.

- Chipped or cracked teeth

- Tooth sensitivity

- Cavities and excessive wear

- Sore jaw muscles

- Gum recession

- A history of multiple crowns and/or root canals

- Trouble chewing certain foods such as steak and bagels

Orchestrating the Bite

One of the big complaints that lets me know someone has a bite issue is that they just "don't know how their bite is supposed to fit together."

Your back teeth are bigger to crush and break down food when you chew, and the muscles in your jaw help make that happen, almost like walnuts in a nutcracker. When everything is working really well, chewing with the back teeth should be effortless. Meanwhile, the teeth in the front of the mouth are smaller and thinner because they're designed to cut food, not crush it. In the front of the mouth you need more of a passive type of bite, where the teeth don't touch with as much intensity.

But most people don't have a perfect bite, one where their teeth and jaw muscles feel comfortable, like they're working together when they close their mouth to chew. In fact, most people often don't realize that their bite is off until they crack a tooth.

Usually, orthodontics primarily straightens the teeth horizontally, but vertically, the teeth may still not have matching peaks and valleys. While aligning the teeth can give you a beautiful-looking smile, often what's needed to correct the bite is a procedure known as **equilibration**. Equilibration is a process of calibrating your bite so that your teeth uniformly contact when your jaws are at rest. It is a gentle procedure that allows your lower teeth to contact your upper teeth very evenly all the way around your mouth.

The three goals of equilibration are:

1. Create equal bilateral bite contacts of the posterior teeth when the muscles are relaxed and the jaw joints are in their proper positions.

2. Have your front teeth help guide and disclude (separate) the back teeth when you move your lower jaw forward or to the side to limit friction and muscle tension while chewing.

3. Eliminate fremitus or mobility of guiding teeth.

The equilibration procedure we utilize uses the Kois Deprogrammer to calibrate the muscles of your jaws, head, and neck to work in symphony with your teeth in a very well-orchestrated way.

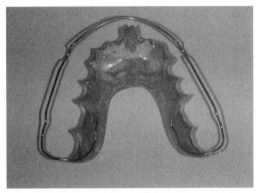

As I mentioned in chapter 3, the deprogrammer is a removable appliance that is worn for at least a week. That time frame allows your jaws to relax and get into a comfortable position following aligner treatment. Then, special paper is inserted into your mouth while you bite down to show contact points; areas of friction; or where there is the potential for chipping, excessive wear, or micromovement. The latter of these, micromovement, can cause gums to recede and be inflamed.

Different colored papers are used to verify different issues with the bite; one paper provides the baseline of your bite on the deprogrammer, which we adjust gradually until your teeth touch (the first point of contact). Once that is identified, then minimal adjustments are made to achieve the three goals previously stated and to polish out the unevenness of your bite while preserving as much tooth structure as possible. Re-mineralizing treatment helps reseal the teeth after polishing for comfort and health.

Added benefits of equilibration include reduced tooth sensitivity, since the teeth fit together better post-treatment. It can also help reduce head and neck pain because wearing the appliance helps to calm the nerve pathways between the head, jaws, and neck, which tests have shown are interconnected.[22]

Adjusting a bite with the Kois Deprogrammer can be complicated and sometimes takes more than one visit. But it's a technology that allows you to be more of a participant in treatment. It permits me to verify your input and see what areas in your mouth I need to adjust. Again, the goal is to make only minimal adjustments to preserve tooth structure while balancing your bite.

Other Bite Technology

Since 2000, I've also used a technique to electronically check the bite on a tooth. Developed by Dr. Robert Kerstein and known as a Tekscan or T-Scan, this instrument provides me with information to use in improving timing and balance of the bite, lessening wear on the teeth, and reducing instances of fractures. The T-scan gives a definitive level of bite pressures, providing more scientific information for more complex cases. It provides more technologically focused insights than patient perceptions or marks on paper. It's especially helpful in identifying teeth that are slightly mobile—something marks on paper won't identify easily or accurately.

There are many tools available to correct a bite and create a beautiful, natural-looking mouth. Sometimes, it's a matter of adjusting surfaces—adding to a tooth/crown or polishing out the rough edge of a tooth or restoration. Sometimes correcting the bite

---

22 W. Y. Lee, J. P. Okeson, and J. Lindroth, "The Relationship Between Forward Head Posture and Temporomandibular Disorders," *Journal of Orofacial Pain* 9, no. 2 (Spring 1995): 161–67, https://www.ncbi.nlm.nih.gov/pubmed/7488986.

requires more complex measures, such as jaw surgery—that may be the case when the skeletal positioning of the upper and lower jaws don't match.

BENEFITS OF A GOOD BITE

- A corrected bite will last longer, cause less discomfort, and result in fewer emergencies.

- Since the teeth fit together as they should, the result is fewer cracked, chipped, and broken teeth or your cosmetic improvements.

- A good bite with aligned teeth is also easier to floss and keep clean.

- Food feels better in the mouth when your bite is aligned, so you're able to eat better foods.

- It just feels great to smile comfortably.

- Perhaps one of the best benefits of a corrected bite is that patients can actually tell later on when their bite is shifting, and then they can draw attention to the need for some changes or alterations. That helps develop a close relationship between dentist and patient for the long-term.

Jackie's Jaws—
No More Pain, A Better Bite

For Jackie, straightening her teeth and balancing her bite eliminated years of problems, and allowed her to chew and live without pain. A balanced bite can help reduce problems that can snowball and ultimately require more-complex treatments. Without having a good, balanced bite, the long-term effects can lead to problems throughout your body that start with wear and tear on the teeth, even to the point of needing to replace teeth.

Replacing teeth often requires implants. Implants are a good solution for missing teeth, but they don't have the proprioceptive (pressure sensing) abilities that natural roots have. Here again, you need a healthy bite before implants are an option. A healthy bite will allow implants to survive longer.

SMILE ON!

How can you take action now to improve your bite?

- Find more ways to relax and not clench or grind your teeth.

- Avoid acidic or highly abrasive toothpaste and foods/drinks that make your teeth more susceptible to wear and cracks.

- Seek out dentists who have special training in bite treatment from places like the Kois Center, The Dawson Academy, or The Spear Center.

- Avoid home-remedy bite guards that are soft and rubbery. They tend to act like "chew toys" and over-stimulate your chewing muscles. They can potentially cause more damage than good.

CHAPTER 8

IMPLANTS CAN MAKE YOU FEEL AS GOOD AS NEW

Adriana came to see me although she was afraid of dentists. She was born and raised in eastern Europe and had some bad experiences with dentistry there. She was a sweet person, but she didn't smile as much she wanted to because of the condition of her teeth. She wanted to improve her smile and to regain her confidence after a divorce.

She came to me originally because she had an implant in the front of her mouth that wasn't done right and was causing irritation on her gums. She also had several teeth that were broken down because of decay or failed root canals. At one point, she had undergone a procedure known as a sinus lift to build bone in her upper jaw, but the area had become infected, leading to some pretty severe problems.

Fortunately, we were able to save the implant. She had several more teeth that needed to be removed, after which we placed implants in those areas as well. Throughout her treatment, we used digital facially generated planning to ensure the teeth were properly guided into place. In other words, we designed where the new teeth would go and then put the implants in the right places for that to happen. The results were seamless.

Today, Adriana's mouth is stable, all her previous problems have been rectified, and she's not afraid to go to the dentist anymore. She knows she has a great smile and her confidence is sky high.

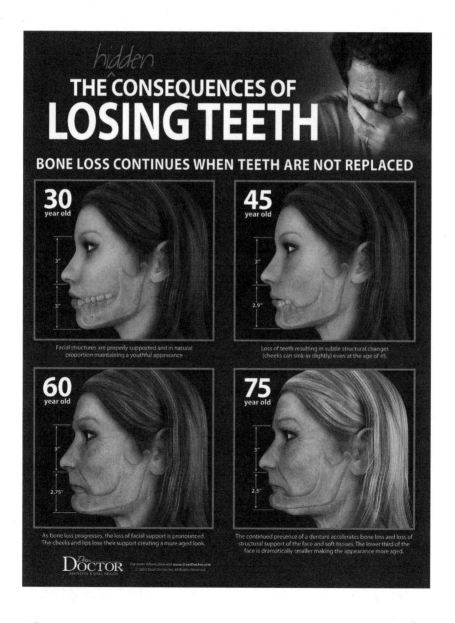

"For years I have gone through numerous cosmetic dentists for whom my case was always too complicated to give me the results I was looking for. Finally, when I first met with Dr. Flax, I literally cried in his office out of the sense of relief of finally finding a specialist who has the knowledge and the skills to deal with my difficult case. Dr. Flax took time to listen to all of my concerns and expectations. … He truly delivered results of my dreams. It feels amazing not needing to hide my smile any more.

"Later, when I was faced with very serious complications from my implant surgery performed by another office, Dr. Flax once again was my saving hero. The same day I contacted Dr. Flax, he immediately treated me and arranged for a medical intervention with his professional colleague, a triple-board certified plastic/ ENT/head and neck surgeon to help my dire situation. After that, Dr. Flax continued to monitor my healing until I was in safe waters again. If it weren't for Dr. Flax, the developing facial disfigurement from the surgery complications would have never been prevented.

"To me, Dr. Flax always has been and always will be the most trusted, the most caring, and the most talented cosmetic genius that dentistry will ever have.

"Dr. Flax has changed my life in so many ways and that's because he gave me the smile I never thought I could have."

—Adriana

See Adriana's progress in the before and after photo section.

Sometimes implants are the best option for rejuvenating a smile—sometimes, they're the only option.

Implants—More Common for Many Reasons

People lose teeth for all kinds of reasons. Yes, teeth can naturally break down over time. But losing a tooth is not always a sign of age or necessarily even poor oral hygiene. Other factors that can lead to tooth loss include diminished bodily health, trauma, eating hard foods, clenching and grinding, or even, as in Adriana's case, poor dentistry.

Many people avoid implantation out of fear of the technology itself. Infection is the number-one reason an implant fails. That's why we take implant dentistry so seriously—when performing a procedure, we put on scrubs just like any surgeon and have a dedicated surgical suite to optimize the final result for our mutual peace of mind.

There are a number of reasons why implants are becoming more common these days:[23]

Longer life span. Today, our population is aging, yet living longer, so many patients are opting to replace missing teeth for more comfort and stability in their bite.

Tooth loss related to aging. Teeth are like other body parts—they can wear out over time. Even teeth that have been stabilized with crowns or other dental treatments can sometimes fail as they age. Often, that's because of trauma caused by your bite.

Bone breakdown. When a tooth is removed from the mouth, enzymes start to break down the bone. Over time, the bone

---

23 Carl Misch, "Rationale for Dental Implants," in *Dental Implant Prosthetics* (St. Louis, MO: Mosby, 2005), 1–15.

wears away. In the first year, most people can lose four millimeters of bone. But it doesn't stop there. Bone continues to break down over time. The more it breaks down, the harder it is to rebuild the bone in that area. The less bone you have, the more grafting has to be done and the less likely that area will look like a natural tooth. In fact, the face can age after losing a tooth—it sinks in once the supporting bone is gone.

To replace fixed bridges. Sometimes, decay in adjacent teeth or gum disease around a fixed bridge can cause it to fail.[24] When that happens, a bridge implant is a viable replacement.[25]

Poor performing dentures. One of the great pioneers of implants, the late Dr. Carl Misch, stated that dentures and removable bridges or partials tend to move around the mouth, which can cause friction and affect the remaining bone and teeth.[26] That can lead to bone breakdown. Dentures and removable bridges or partials just spread problems around in the mouth and create new ones, instead of focusing on the problem itself—a missing tooth.

Emotional loss. People often feel that losing a tooth is the beginning of the end. Losing a tooth is more than a physical change in the body. It's an emotional loss that can cause

---

24 S. Palmqvist and B. Swartz, "Artificial Crowns and Fixed Partial Dentures 18 to 23 Years After Placement," *The International Journal of Prosthodontics* 6, no. 3 (May–June 1993): 279–85, https://www.ncbi.nlm.nih.gov/pubmed/8397697.

25 G.F. Priest, "Failure Rates of Restorations for Single-tooth Replacement," The International Journal of Prosthodontics 9, no. 1 (January–February 1996): 38–45, https://www.ncbi.nlm.nih.gov/pubmed/8630176.

26 Carl Misch, "The Hidden Consequences of Losing Teeth: How Dental Implants Stop Gradual Bone Loss and Replace Teeth," *Dear Doctor Dentistry & Oral Health*, accessed March 20 2019, www.deardoctor.com/articles/hidden-consequences-of-losing-teeth.

patients to experience grief. It reminds them of what their parents may have gone through in losing some or all of their teeth. They may have seen a parent's dentures soaking in a glass next to the bed. They may even experience fear in the memory of seeing their parents without their teeth in.

Despite that, they may end up getting dentures, but then won't wear them because they're not comfortable, they move around, or they make it too difficult to properly chew food. Sometimes, it's because the patient has trouble adjusting to their new mouth. Often, it's because the dentures weren't made right or they don't fit correctly. YouTube has plenty of videos of people who are enjoying themselves at a wedding or event or even parachuting—but they open their mouth to smile and their denture falls out.

Some people almost feel like losing a tooth makes them disabled or handicapped in some way. They're like "oral invalids" or a "dental cripple." Even the stigma of having to purchase dental adhesive can be shocking to them. They're so embarrassed by the idea of wearing an "oral wig" that it affects their ability to work with others or seek career advancement, and they just begin to age. The loss of three or four teeth can become noticeable.

Over time, ill-fitting dentures can end up causing nutritional problems—if it becomes too difficult to properly chew, they end up eating nothing but soft foods. In a world trending toward healthier eating, people with ill-fitting dentures can have trouble keeping up. Denture wearers may even become more isolated—they may stop socializing because they don't feel confident talking to people or eating in public.

But here's the really sad part: The longer the person waits, the worse the situation gets. Putting off treatment out of a fear of going to the dentist or out of fear over the implant procedure itself only promotes more bone loss.

The earlier you deal with tooth loss, the younger we can keep you and the more natural the final result will be.

The Implant Procedure

Let me share with you what it's like to actually go through the process of getting an implant. As you read this, remember that you're in the hands of professionals who have empathy for your situation and want to use their experience and expertise to help you get back a beautiful—and functional—smile.

Performing an implant procedure begins with a plan for what the end result will be. That means knowing exactly where the teeth are supposed to fit your bite and how they will fit your face. The implants should not only function just like natural teeth, they should also restore facial contours. The whole goal is for you to be comfortable with the teeth restored, but to also be able to chew, smile, and speak over a lifetime.

Starting with the end in mind, we take digital images using the CBCT, which produces 3-D images of the structures of your head and neck. The images the CBCT produces show all the remaining teeth in your mouth and how much bone is left where you have missing teeth. Impressions of your mouth are also taken, often using the digital scanner, and we take digital photos of your mouth and face to help aesthetically and architecturally plan where the tooth or teeth are to be placed. Digital overlays from the data gathered reveal gaps in the bone and allow us to plan the ideal size and position of each implant.

Once all the information about your mouth and health is gathered, we create a treatment plan. During that planning, if a patient says, "I just want to look like I did before," I ask them to bring in pictures of a happy moment so we can see how their teeth looked when they smiled. That also helps shape the treatment plan.

The treatment plan includes determining whether there is enough bone to support the implants and keep them rigid for long-term health. Depending on the complexity of the case, for instance, areas that need extra grafting, the patient may be referred to a specialist. But even cases requiring as many as five teeth can often be handled in our office. It really comes down to the amount of bone that has been lost. Major amounts of missing bone may be grafted by a specialist, who may be better equipped to build back the bone. In some of those cases, the specialist also places the implant.

Before I go any further, let me take a minute to explain bone grafting.

When a tooth is lost or extracted from the mouth, the bone of the jaw where the tooth was located can recede—it's almost like creating a sinkhole after a tree and its roots are removed. Where the tree was located, the ground begins to sink in.

To compensate for this, a bone (the graft) can be placed into the area where the tooth is removed to solidify the area, help with healing, and preserve the volume and density of the bone so that an implant can be placed. That's why implants should be considered very early in a treatment plan when there's a risk that a tooth is coming out—because sometimes the implant can be placed at the same time as the extraction.

At the time a tooth is removed, the amount of remaining bone is monitored because the goal is to preserve as much bone as possible. If there is enough bone when the tooth is removed, or if only a small amount of bone must be added, then often the implant is placed at that time. In fact, the ideal situation is to place the implant when the tooth is removed, for a number of reasons, including reducing bone recession and because healing can occur concurrently with the tooth removal.

There are two different types of bone grafts—either allograft or autograft. **Allograft** is a graft made of sterilized cadaver bone. The safety of allografts is well documented, and protocols are strictly managed. **Autograft** is a graft using the patient's own bone, typically taken from some area of the mouth, usually where your wisdom teeth previously existed, or, rarely, taken from the patient's hip for major jaw augmentation. With today's technologies in bioengineering to rebuild tissue, we have the ability to use a patient's own natural growth factors to enhance the vitality of the graft. We simply take a small blood sample, spin it down, extract the growth factors, and then mix them in with a bone graft to get a better result. If a graft is needed, it may take three to four months, or more, to heal before the implant is placed. Once there is enough bone, then the size of the implant is determined—with that information, the trajectory or direction of the implant is determined.

Every time we place an implant, my team and I scrub and gown to decrease the risk of infection—we take it as seriously as any other surgery. The procedure involves making a small incision in the gum to create room for the implant, and sometimes to expand the bone.

Implants are tiny, prosthetic posts made of titanium or titanium alloy, which does not irritate the soft tissue of the mouth. Some newer breeds of implants are being made of zirconia—the same type of zirconia used for hip replacements. This advancement we believe will serve people who want a metal-free solution or who, because of their gums, are hoping to have a more esthetic result. At this point in time, the jury is still out on the use of zirconia, although some dentists have found it to be extremely reliable for replacing one or two teeth, leaving titanium for cases involving more teeth.

If there's enough bone to proceed without grafting, then the implant or post is placed into the bone of the jaw, with the top surface resting at approximately bone level, usually three to four millimeters below the gumline. A small screw is placed into the implant to cover it and to help create an ideal shape for the gum to heal to.

After the implant is placed, the incision is closed up and then we check on your progress over the next three to four months. The implant takes several months to fuse to the bone, a process known as **osseointegration**. Under normal circumstances where there's enough bone, the density of the bone is very healthy, and little or no grafting was done, osseointegration takes around three months. Depending on the circumstances, the entire implant procedure, from tooth removal to placing the crown, can take six to nine months to complete. Considering that a natural tooth takes nine to ten years to grow, replacing a tooth that is lost with a procedure that takes six to nine months is a significant improvement.

After the implant fuses, then the crown is designed. The crown is the tooth part of the implant. It is designed to fit the space and look and function like the tooth it is replacing.

Making Your Implant Look Like a Tooth—and Last Longer

Once the implant is placed, if the space shows in your smile, we may place a temporary crown over the implant just to enhance your appearance. The quantity and quality of the bone and location of the tooth determines whether a temporary is placed while waiting for the implant to heal. In the back of your mouth, the temporary is not designed to withstand heavier bite forces and is not intended to function as the final crown will. Temporaries can also disturb the healing of the implant, so they are not ideal for every case. While this part of the procedure is not appropriate for all implants, the beauty of it is that it helps make for pristine tissue when it's time to make the impression for the final crown. That helps produce a very accurate crown.

There are two types of implant crowns: screw retained and cement retained. With a **screw-retained** implant, a screw actually holds the crown to the implant. With a **cement-retained** one, a small component known as an abutment is screwed onto the implant, then the crown is cemented onto the abutment. There are advantages to each type.

The primary advantage of the screw retained is reversibility. Screw-retained implants can give you peace of mind if there's a concern about something going awry. It may also be a better option when there is limited room for the crown.

The advantage of the cement-retained implant is that it is can be a better looking crown, since there is no screw access hole, and it is more resistant to fracture. One disadvantage, however, is that the cement used to attach the crown to the abutment can sometimes irritate the gums—that's why a perfectly fitting crown is so important.

An important point to consider: Implants don't have shock-absorbing capabilities, so while they look nice and function well, they're not exactly like a natural tooth. Teeth are made of natural material; implants are made of foreign material like titanium and zirconia. Teeth are naturally connected to the bone by fiber-like tissues that surround the roots of the tooth. Those roots are also surrounded by a sack of fluid that acts like a "shock absorber." The biology of a natural tooth gives your brain feedback on how much bite pressure you can use—it lets you know how hard or soft you can chew. Plus, those natural, fiber-like tissues and the sack of fluid give the tooth a more natural feel. Since implants fuse to the bone, there is no shock-absorbing effect. As a result, you lose the feedback to your brain on how much pressure to apply when you chew.

Even though there is no shock absorber, you don't feel pain with implants. But without the feedback mechanism, it's possible to overload the bone in some cases. In addition, the density of the bone in the upper and lower jaws is different: the lower jaw bone is denser, while the upper is spongier or softer. It's like comparing oak to balsa wood.

Fine-tuning the bite in the final crown can make it more rigid by eliminating lateral or side-to-side chewing forces that can affect the performance of an implant and potentially cause it to break down. Implants actually tend to do very well with teeth that have vertical chewing forces—those teeth are in the back of the mouth. Implants also work in the front teeth, where a tooth needs to be replaced for esthetics, but because the chewing forces are more lateral, the bone is thinner, and the roots are shorter, then the bite must be made more passive (i.e., have lighter forces).

When there is concern about damage to an implant because of bite forces or clenching and grinding, a nighttime bite appliance may also be prescribed. This appliance is a bite guard that becomes the shock absorber, taking the brunt of the torque and pressure on the teeth and decreasing the friction that can cause the implant to break down. This is a strategy supported in recent literature.[27]

---

27   B.R. Chrcanovic et al., "Bruxism and Dental Implant Failures: A Multilevel Mixed Effects Parametric Survival Analysis Approach," *Journal of Oral Rehabilitation* 43, no. 11 (November 2016): 813–23, https://doi.org/10.1111/joor.12431.

The Modern Improvement for Dentures

For many years, dentures have been a common solution to replace multiple teeth. Although the stories about George Washington's wooden teeth are myth, he did wear different sets of dentures made of various materials, including gold, lead, ivory, and even human teeth.[28]

As mentioned previously, dentures and removable bridges or partials often move around the mouth, leading to friction that negatively impacts remaining bone and teeth and can even lead to bone breakdown. Dentures and removable bridges or partials just create more problems in the mouth and don't really address the real problem—a missing tooth.

Instead of a "tooth wig" to coverup and loosely replace the missing teeth, implants can:

Improve the retention and stability of a denture (implant assisted "overdentures")

Completely retain the replacement of the teeth as a bridge would since the teeth are cemented on or screwed into the implants (implant retained and supported)

Both of these implant types—implant assisted "overdentures" and implant retained and supported—are sophisticated treatments that we do in collaboration with a specialized lab technician and occasionally a surgeon.

---

28 "Wooden Teeth Myth," The Fred W. Smith National Library for the Study of George Washington, *George Washington's Mount Vernon*, accessed March 20, 2019, www.mountvernon.org/library/digitalhistory/digital-encyclopedia/article/wooden-teeth-myth.

With today's enhanced digital technology and bioengineering materials, there are also solutions for replacing multiple teeth in one day. Commonly known as "Same-Day Teeth," "Teeth In A Day," or other similar names, this intensive procedure involves removing the teeth, cleaning up the bone, placing multiple implants, and then placing a one-piece prosthesis on the implants, essentially like a permanent bridge. The prosthesis is a prototype to wear while you heal and the implants integrate into the bone. The huge benefit is that you immediately get to smile and chew as you have been dreaming of for years without the embarrassment of missing or loose teeth. The recommended healing time to stabilize the bone and implants is usually six to twelve months. Once everything is healed and stabilized, a stronger, more permanent titanium or zirconia supported "hybrid bridge" is designed and placed in your mouth.

Single implants are cleaned and flossed just like natural teeth. Multiple implants splinted together must be flossed underneath, like a bridge—floss must be carefully threaded between the porcelain crowns and the gums. A water irrigator is also a good tool to have when cleaning multiple implants that are splinted or bridged together.

A New Outlook for Adriana

As you can see, there's a lot involved in determining whether an implant is the best solution. For Adriana, implants were the only solution—but ideal for giving her a happier, healthier future.

When it comes to implants, being proactive is key. The more proactive you are, the better the chance that the treatment will be easier. Plus, the more complicated the treatment, the higher the cost. For instance, whether an implant can be placed at the time a tooth is extracted may not be known until the tooth comes out, but the longer you wait, the greater the chance that the bone will be severely broken down. That may then require grafting before an implant can be done.

While implants are a very good option for replacing teeth, nothing compares to having your natural teeth in your mouth. A mouthful of healthy, strong teeth gives you the ability to chew well, providing the right nutrition to maintain your long-term health and appearance.

SMILE ON!

What you can do now about implants:

- Don't let a diseased tooth stay in your mouth too long.

- Make sure your treatment includes 3-D digital planning.

- Find a dentist who is experienced in not only placing implants but also in managing your gums and bite so the implant has a greater chance of survival.

WELLNESS IS THE KEY TO HELPING THE MOUTH AND BODY SYNERGIZE

Kevin initially came to see me with multiple toothaches. He was overweight and fearful about going to the dentist. He had generalized decay and gum infection, which had fortunately not extended deep into his bone. That allowed us to treat him conservatively. His bite was also a factor; he was clenching very hard, which was related to sleep apnea, or trouble breathing during sleep—when breathing is difficult at night, the teeth can clench to keep the airway open.

Since Kevin wasn't taking care of his gums, he wasn't able to eat nutritious foods, and his heart health was suffering. He had high blood pressure and was definitely at high risk for heart disease. In fact, his weight put him at risk for a whole slew of health problems. During treatment planning, I even spoke to his physician, who was concerned about the state of Kevin's health, who was only age thirty at the time.

We performed deep gum treatments on Kevin, including gum irrigation, and targeted antibiotic therapy. We sampled his plaque and found that the biofilm from his teeth had bad bacteria that made his mouth acidic enough to decalcify (soften) his teeth and make him more prone to gum infection. That helped us target what kind of antibiotic to prescribe for him, and the medication helped speed up the healing process. He also needed root canals, which were provided by a specialist. Then, we balanced his bite using the Kois Deprogrammer (as discussed in chapter 7). With the bacteria and bite under control, we whitened his teeth and placed two crowns on teeth that were severely decayed. We also bonded other teeth to repair smaller areas of decay.

A critical step in Kevin's treatment was changing the acidity of his mouth—since the pH of his mouth was too low, contributing to the breakdown of his teeth. Low pH can cause the calcium and phosphate in your mouth to move out of the teeth and make them weaker. By raising the pH of his mouth with CariFree products, we were able to improve his mouth to undergo normal dental procedures while also strengthening his teeth. Cavities in the early stages of development, where the decay is only appearing on the outer layer of the enamel, can often be reversed with re-mineralization, which strengthens the calcium and phosphate of teeth. Such treatments can also save the patient money over bonding and can even prevent future cavities.

Once we resolved his bite and gum issues and repaired his teeth, he continued on a good preventive program. Besides brushing and flossing, he now uses a special toothpaste to help re-mineralize his teeth. In addition, we prescribed a nighttime bite guard for Kevin to decrease the potential damage to his teeth from clenching during sleep.

Many of Kevin's problems with his overall health were the result of the breakdown of this oral health.

Post-treatment, his mouth feels better, he feels better, he's watching what he eats, and he's lost nearly one hundred pounds. He has more energy—he looks and moves like a different man.

"Dr. Hugh Flax and his team are amazing! I have always hated visiting the dentist, but no longer. He and his staff are always so friendly and professional every time I visit. I would highly recommend him to anyone that struggles with visiting the dentist."

—**Kevin**

See Kevin's progress in the before and after photo section.

Mouth and Body—There Is a Connection

There is a bidirectional connection between the mouth and the body; when your mouth and body synergize, your body becomes much healthier. But when the mouth has breakdown or disease, it can affect the rest of your body.

As I mentioned in chapter 1, research has found a link between oral inflammation and infection and health problems in other areas of the body, such as heart disease, diabetes, and premature birth or low-birth-weight babies.[29]

To understand how that's possible, let me explain how it's all connected. When you have acids in your mouth—either because of poor oral hygiene, an unhealthy diet (with acidic foods and drinks), conditions such as GERD or bulimia, or other reasons—you start

---

29   Mayo Clinic Staff, "Oral Health: A Window to Your Overall Health," *Mayo Clinic*, November 1, 2018, accessed February 5, 2019, www.mayoclinic.org/healthy-lifestyle/adult-health/in-depth/dental/art-20047475%20--.

to lose calcium and phosphate on your teeth, which makes them weaker. Harmful bacteria can begin to build up in such an environment, making your gums more prone to infection. If your teeth and gums aren't healthy, they start to break down and become inflamed. That inflammation signals your body's immune system to attack the bacteria in an effort to bring the situation under control. If that doesn't happen, then your gums (and more importantly your supporting bone) continue to break down and you develop **periodontitis**, disease of the bone and gums.

Where things go really wrong, however, is when the inflammation from your gums spreads to other areas of your body. Here are some of the problems that can occur as a result:

Heart disease. Infection in the gums can eventually cause inflammation in the blood vessels. A substance called C reactive protein (CRP) is created by the liver and binds to the white blood cells that try to fight the infection. Those blood vessels can become almost sticky, catching and holding onto blood cells to cause thickening of the arteries. That can increase your blood pressure, which then places pressure on your heart. If any of the plaque that builds up in those thicker arteries breaks loose and travels to the heart or brain, they can cause a heart attack or stroke. The Mayo Clinic has reported that more than 90 percent of patients with heart disease also have gum disease, perhaps in part because the two conditions are also linked by risk factors such as smoking, unhealthy eating, and being overweight.[30]

Diabetes. There is a two-way connection when it comes to oral health and diabetes. When your mouth is unhealthy

30   Mayo Clinic Staff, op. cit., "Oral Health: A Window to Your Overall Health."

and you're not able to eat properly, your blood sugar goes up because inflammation in your mouth makes it harder for your body to control it. At that point, you have a higher risk of having diabetes because high blood sugar makes it easier for infection to take hold—including in your gums. Gum disease tends to be more frequent and severe when people have diabetes. The good news is that controlling one tends to control the other—keeping the mouth healthy can help control diabetes, and keeping blood sugar under control can help keep your gums healthy.[31]

Problems with pregnancy. Early or low-weight babies can have problems ranging from lung and heart development conditions to learning disorders. Periodontitis (gum disease) in the mother—potentially caused by the changes in hormones during pregnancy—may interfere with the development of a fetus in the womb.

Smoking and oral health. Smoking can cause problems in the mouth as well as in other areas of the body. Since nicotine causes the blood vessels to constrict, it can interfere with the gums' ability to ward off infection.[32]

Arthritis, COPD, obesity, osteoporosis. Other connections are being made between rheumatoid arthritis (reducing gum inflammation can reduce arthritis pain), lung conditions (periodontal disease may worsen chronic obstructive pulmonary disease or COPD), and obesity (higher levels of body fat may cause gum disease to progress more rapidly).

---

31 Ibid.

32 Joanne Barker, "Oral Health: The Mouth-Body Connection," *WebMD*, January 4, 2012, accessed February 24, 2019, www.webmd.com/oral-health/features/oral-health-the-mouth-body-connection#1.

The connection to osteoporosis is somewhat controversial, but some in the medical profession theorize that bone breakdown in the mouth could trigger more bone breakdown throughout the body.

There are many links now being made between oral health and overall health. One study found that people that had gum disease were as much as 40 percent more likely to also have a chronic condition.[33] Thankfully, medical and dental professionals are beginning to recognize the symptoms and working together to manage or reverse the problems.

Improving Your Health

So, good oral health can make a world of difference in your overall health. When you take better care of your mouth, you have a better chance of taking care of your body and keeping away the inflammation and bacteria that can get into your bloodstream and produce infection throughout your body. Here are some ways to do that.

Brush and floss. Brushing your teeth at least twice a day and flossing daily are two easy to implement steps to improving your oral and overall health.

Eat healthy. Improve your nutrition by eating a healthy diet and avoiding acidic foods and drinks such as carbonated beverages and lemons.

Improve your pH levels. Improving the pH in your mouth decreases its acidity. That can keep your teeth strong and also improve the acidity in your body. When the acidity in your body increases, you become more prone to inflammation, which can lead to other diseases.

---

33   Mayo Clinic Staff, op. cit., "Oral Health: A Window to Your Overall Health."

Avoid tobacco use. That means not just cigarettes but chewing tobacco and vaping. The chemicals from those products combined with the heat in your mouth lowers your body's resistance and makes you more prone to having gum infections. Tobacco products and vaping also disturb the soft tissues in the mouth and make you more prone to soft tissue diseases, including oral cancer.

Get better sleep. Sleep is also an important part of oral health. Breathing is not an option—you can't live without it. Yet people with sleep apnea stop breathing in their sleep repeatedly. When a person stops breathing repeatedly because of sleep apnea, they can begin to lack oxygen. That can cause your cardiovascular system to work harder and potentially increase your chances of a heart attack. A body that is low on oxygen doesn't perform as well. Better sleep means a better oxygenated body. The bottom graphic on the next page depicts the likelihood of having obstructive sleep apnea (OSA) with a given medical condition. On the right side are the studies supporting these numbers. In other words, these statistics show that, if you have one of these conditions, you may have OSA as a concurrent condition. Bottom line: If you have bad medical problems, there's a high chance that OSA is part of the problem. There is also a causal link between sleep-disordered breathing and insulin resistance in adult onset diabetes.[34] While dentists cannot diagnose OSA, they do have an obligation to be health advocates, and subsequently, a responsibility to share the risks of a disease impli-

---

34   Tasali, Esra MD, et al. "Sleep Disordered Breathing and the current epidemic of obesity: Consequence or contributing factor.": Am J respir Crit Care Med. 2002;165: 562-563.

cated in many of the leading causes of death. Studies have shown that you have a three times higher chance of heart attack with OSA than if you are overweight or have high blood pressure.[35]

Independant Predictors for Risk of Future M.I. ;

Risk Factor	Odds Ratio
Standard	1.0
Overweight	7.1
Hypertension	7.8
Smoking	11.1
OSA	23.3

Hypertension	30%	Nieto-JAMA 2000
Drug Resistant Hypertension	83%	Logan-Hypertension 2001
Chronic Heart Failure (40%C 30%O)	76%	Oldenburg-Eur J Heart Failure
Congestive Heart Failure	85%	Jiang-Journal of Cardiac Failure 2007
Atrial Fibrillation	49%	Gami-Nat Clin Pract Cardiovasc Med 2005
Ischemic Heart Disease	38%	Mooe-Am J Respir Crit Care Med 2001
Stroke	92%	NorAdina-Singapore Med J 2006
Medically Refractory Epilepsy	33%	Malow-Neurology 2000
Metabolic Syndrome	50%	Ambrosetti-J Cardiovasc Med 2006
Type II Diabetes	48%	Einhorn-Endocr Pract. 2007
Obese Diabetes	70%	Brooks-J Clin Endocrinol Metab 1994
Morbid Obesity Male 90% Female	50%	Fritscher-Obes Surg 2007
GERD (same for snoring as OSA)	60%	Valipour-Chest 2002

---

35   Hung et. al., "Association of sleep apnea with myocardial infarction in men," Lancet Aug. 4, 1990; 336 (8710): 261-4

Less-Obvious Effects of Lack of Sleep

Besides feeling groggy and lethargic, below-average sleep duration and quality lead to other, less-obvious or even hidden challenges:

Clenching, leading to tooth damage. When you stop breathing during sleep, your jaws automatically clench as a way of opening up your airway. Clenching can cause the teeth and bone to break down over time. When I see broken teeth in someone's mouth during an exam, I begin asking questions to see if we're looking a problem with sleep apnea.

Fatigue, which can affect the immune system, the brain, and your mental health. Poor sleep quantity and quality cause your body to lack the refreshment and fatigue reversal that it craves, which affects your immune function, your memory, and your psychological well-being. When you can sleep longer, your body is able to repair itself and that tends to make you less prone to having problems, such as gum infections.

Food cravings, leading to weight gain. A body deprived of sleep also craves food. When you get less sleep, your body secretes chemicals from the pituitary gland that causes you to feel like you're hungry. All that extra eating can make you more obese, which can lead to other health problems, such as diabetes and heart disease.

Snoring—not just for adults. Pediatric snoring is not kids' stuff. Snoring is one of the key symptoms of sleep apnea, which is not just a problem found in adults. In children, sleep problems are sometimes the result of jaw and teeth development. Breathing is greatly affected by the positions of the jaws and the size of the oral cavity. If a child's mouth is not large enough, their tongue tends to struggle with its position. That can lead to crowding in the mouth and problems with breathing and sleep apnea. When a child loses sleep over time, or they are deprived of oxygen because of a blockage in their airway due to the tongue not having enough room, then their brain does not develop as well. Constant disruptions during sleep can interrupt the release of certain hormones that children need during development. They can end up have memory problems, learning problems, poor performance in school, lower IQs, and even be diagnosed as having attention deficit disorder (ADD). Worse still, a doctor or pediatrician may start medicating them for ADD or even prescribe a growth hormone—when all the child really needs is to be able to breathe better and sleep well.

The best solution is creating enough room inside their mouth for their tongue to rest comfortably, so that it doesn't fall back in their throat during sleep and block the airway.

Unfortunately, when untreated, these problems tend to have a cumulative, cascading effect, leading to many adult problems such as cardiovascular problems, brain function, and even problems operating machinery at work or driving a vehicle.

Dentists are in the best position to notice these types of problems. They're more equipped in many ways to be a good adjunct or bidirectional referral source with physicians, pediatricians, and adult primary caregivers. And the earlier we deal with these problems, the better the chance of a person having a happier, healthier life. When we see problems in children, we always recommend a pediatric ENT and/or orthodontist to rectify these matters as proactively as possible.

Better Tools to Treat Gum Disease and Tooth Decay

In medicine, precise targeted tests are done to identify risk factors, levels of bacteria, or levels of chemicals in your bloodstream. Dentistry is similar to medicine because it sometimes requires testing that's outside the range of what dentists usually do to diagnose problems. We get a broader spectrum of information by running those tests.

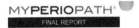

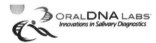

Smith, Jane	Ordering Provider (10000022)	Sample Information
Date Of Birth: 10/11/1941 Gender: Female	Hugh Flax DDS 1100 Lake Hearn Dr Ste 440 Atlanta, GA 30342 404-255-9080	Accession: 30052429 Received: 02/12/2014 11:29 Specimen: Oral Rinse Reported: 02/14/2014 14:55 Collected: 02/06/2014 Printed: 02/14/2014 14:56

Result: POSITIVE - 4 PATHOGENIC BACTERIA REPORTED ABOVE THRESHOLD [Td][Fn][Pm][Ec]
Bacterial Risk: HIGH - Strong evidence of increased risk for attachment loss

Legend
— = Pathogen Load Threshold*
DL = Detection Limit

Result Interpretation: Periodontal disease is caused by specific, or groups of specific bacteria. Threshold levels represent the concentration above which patients are generally at increased risk for attachment loss. Bacterial levels should be considered collectively and in context with clinical signs and other risk factors.

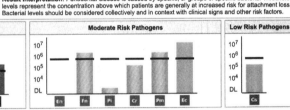

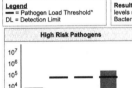

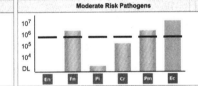

	Pathogen	Result	Clinical Significance
Td	Treponema denticola	High	Very strong association with PD: invasive in cooperation with other bacteria. Usually seen in combination with other bacteria.
Fn	Fusobacterium nucleatum/periodonticum	High	Strong association with PD: adherence properties to several oral pathogens; often seen in refractory disease.
Pm	Peptostreptococcus (Micromonas) micros	High	Moderate association with PD: detected in higher numbers at sites of active disease.
Ec	Eikenella corrodens	High	Moderate association with PD: Found more frequently in active sites of disease; often seen in refractory disease.
Aa	Aggregatibacter actinomycetemcomitans	Low	Very strong association with PD: Transmittable, tissue invasive, and pathogenic at relatively low bacterial counts. Associated with aggressive forms of disease.
Tf	Tannerella forsythia	Low	Very strong association with PD: common pathogen associated with refractory periodontitis. Strongly related to increasing pocket depths.
Pi	Prevotella intermedia	Low	Strong association with PD: virulent properties similar to Pg; often seen in refractory disease.
Cr	Campylobacter rectus	Low	Moderate association with development of PD: usually found in combination with other suspected pathogens in refractory disease.
Cs	Capnocytophaga species (gingavalis,ochracea,sputigena)	Low	Some association with PD: Frequently found in gingivitis. Often found in association with other periodontal pathogens. May increase temporarily following active therapy.

Not Detected: (Pg) Porphyromonas gingivalis, (En) Eubacterium nodatum

Additional information is available from MyOralDNA.com on Interpreting Results

Methodology: Genomic DNA is extracted from the submitted sample and tested for 13 bacteria associated with periodontal disease. The bacteria are tested by polymerase chain reaction (PCR) amplification followed by fluorescent endpoint detection of sample bacterial concentrations (e.g. 10^3 = 1000 bacteria copies per amplified reaction). *Modified from: Microbiological goals of periodontal therapy; Periodontology 2000, Vol. 42, 2006, 180-218. **Disclaimer:** 1. OralDNA is not liable for any outcomes arising from clinician's treatment protocols and decisions. Dentists should consult with a periodontist or patient's physician when infections are advanced or as indicated by patient's medical condition. 2. OralDNA is not responsible for inaccurate test results due to poor sample collection. 3. This test was developed and its performance characteristics determined by OralDNA Labs pursuant to CLIA requirements. It has not been cleared or approved by the U.S. Food and Drug Administration. The FDA has determined that such clearance or approval is not necessary. 4. MyPerioPath collection should occur before rinsing with antimicrobials (as it may temporarily reduce bacterial quantity).

OralDNA Labs, A Service of Access Genetics, LLC, 7400 Flying Cloud Drive, Eden Prairie, MN 55344   855-ORALDNA: Fax: 952-767-0446 www.oraldna.com
Medical Director: Ronald McGlennen, MD   Page 1 of 3

Any time the signs of gum disease exist (bone loss, bleeding, tooth mobility), we use a test called OralDNA. It helps us to diagnose gum disease and risk factors faster than we were able to in the past. It allows us to identify hidden and specific bacteria that can threaten the mouth and the systemic health of the body. We conduct an OralDNA test before we start treatment to get a baseline of the bacteria that we're dealing with, and whether those bacteria are high or low risk.

High-risk bacteria tend to break down the bone more quickly and they often tend to be what are known as nonaerobic bacteria. They thrive without oxygen and tend to be deeper under the gums where the tissue is broken down. These bacteria need to be targeted. When tests reveal the presence of these bacteria, the patient is put on antibiotics. That's all done before removing the physical irritants in the gums, such as calculus and plaque. Patients are also taught how to manage the problems with their gums.

Once treatment is complete, and the patient has healed, the OralDNA tests are run again to determine whether the bacteria in question is below the threshold for causing further damage.

Potential complications that may affect the healing and prognosis of resolving gum disease include:

- **Higher stress levels that lower immunity.** Unfortunately, when some people are exposed to more stress, the levels of cortisol (the stress hormone) in their body increase to help the body cope. Too much cortisol can cause a spike in viruses or in certain bacteria—and then gum disease returns. It's almost like a thermostat that gets cranked up way beyond normal or what's comfortable. Whenever the body's immune system breaks down, gums and bone become more prone to permanent damage.

- **Chronic gum disease.** Some patients have a problem called **periodontosis**, where the gum problem never really resolves itself. This refractory problem often has multiple causes, including genetics. Usually a specialist is needed to treat and monitor this condition.

To combat tooth decay, in 2003, my practice adopted a model known as Caries Management by Risk Assessment (CAMBRA), which is an evidence-based approach that looks at the risk factors and how those translate to the chance of decay.[36]

For instance, if the CAMBRA identifies someone as low risk, then there's a 23 percent chance of them getting new cavities within a year. Whereas a patient who is high risk has an 88 percent higher chance of getting tooth decay. The more risk factors you have, the more you get placed into the extreme risk category. By identifying those risks, we can decide whether we should try to re-mineralize your teeth using different products or, if you're at a high risk—a small cavity is going to get bigger no matter what—then we go ahead and treat it.[37]

---

36 John D. B. Featherstone, "The Caries Balance: Contributing Factors and Early Detection," *Journal of the California Dental Association* 31, no. 2 (February 2003): 129–33, https://ozonewithoutborders.ngo/wp-content/uploads/2017/07/caries-balance.pdf.

37 Douglas A. Young, John D. B. Featherstone, Jon R. Roth, "Curing the Silent Epidemic: Caries Management in the 21st Century and Beyond," *Journal of the California Dental Association* 35, no. 10 (October 2007): 681-.85, https://www.researchgate.net/publication/5804278_Curing_the_silent_epidemic_Caries_management_in_the_21st_century_and_beyond; JDB Featherstone and B. W. Chaffee, "The Evidence for Caries Management by Risk Assessment (CAMBRA)," *Advances in Dental Research* 29, no. 1 (February 2018): 9–14, https://doi.org/10.1177/0022034517736500.

Habits and conditions that might put you in the high-risk category include:

- smoking

- bulimia

- acid reflux

- reduced salivary flow

Dry mouth can lower pH in your mouth and eliminate antibodies that help keep bad bacteria in check. Some causes of dry mouth include head and neck radiation therapy, which can cause salivary gland dysfunction, and Sjögren's syndrome, which is a disorder of the immune system that affects the salivary and tear glands. Medically prescribed drugs can also cause dry mouth. Illicit drugs such as methamphetamine, marijuana, cocaine, and ecstasy cause a dramatic decrease in salivary flow, making the teeth extremely prone to decay. These drugs can also cause people to crave the wrong foods and drinks, including carbonated beverages and an excess of alcoholic beverages.

Here are a couple of charts to help you control pH with the food and drinks you consume.

WATER BRAND	ACID LEVELS	
Alkalized Ionized Water	9.5 to 11.5	
Tap Water	7.00 (Neutral)	
Penta Water	4.0	
Distilled Water	4.0	
Purified Water	4.0	
Aquafina (Pepsi)	4.0	
Dasani (Coke)	4.0	
Glaceau Fruit Water	4.0	
Le Blue Water	4.0	
Metro Mint Water	4.0	
Pellegrino	4.0	
Perrier	4.0	
Smart Water	4.0	
Vitamin Water	4.0	
Purified and Reverse Osmosis Water	4.5-6.0 (Depending on Source)	
IceAge Glacial Water	4.5	
Appalachian Springs Water	5.0	
Poland Springs Water	5.0	Low = BAD
Pure American Water	5.5	7.0 = Neutral
Dannon Spring Water	5.5	Over 7.0 = GOOD
Arrowhead Water	7.0	
Crystal Geyser Water	7.0	
Deer Park Water	7.0	
Eldorado Springs Water	7.0	
Supermarket Spring Water	7.0	
Biota Water	7.5	
Fiji Water	7.5	
Whole Foods 365 Water	7.5	
Zephyr Hills Water	7.5	
Eden Springs Water	7.9	
Deep Rock Water	8.0	
Evamore Water	8.0	
Fiji Water	7.5	
Alkalized Ionized Water	9.5 to 11.2	

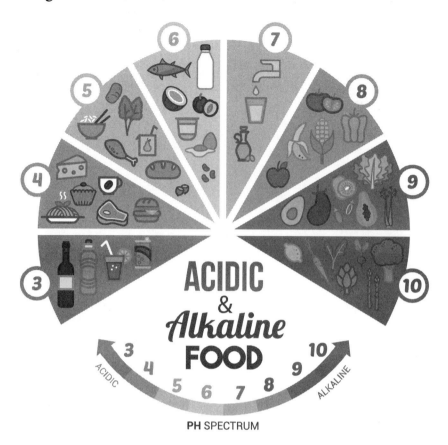

PH SPECTRUM

Dentistry used to take a pretty simplified view of mouth health—
if you brushed and flossed you wouldn't get cavities. Today, we know
that the quality and quantity of the saliva are also important, because
that can determine whether a mouth is too acidic, which can lead to
decaying conditions. The bottom line is that the environment of the
mouth must be controlled.

In addition to the CariFree products I've mentioned, there are
other treatments that can help reverse some gum problems. For
instance, using xylitol gum is another treatment that might be recommended. When you're actively trying to improve the oral environment and make it more neutral, the calcium and phosphate can
return to the tooth and bacteria won't thrive, which helps your body
rebalance itself.

The Root Canal Controversy

There is some controversy these days about root canals. There's a lot of finger pointing to root canals as being the cause of cancer or other diseases that occur in other areas of the body. But there are many assumptions in that claim and no real scientific evidence. For instance, there's misinformation out there about root canals leaving a diseased—and deceased—tooth in the mouth. That's simply not true—root canals—when done correctly—can regenerate healthy bone and nerves and blood supply around a tooth.

Root canals are sometimes necessary, but just like any medical procedure, there are no 100 percent guarantees. Now, I'm not saying every root canal is good. What I am saying is that bad root canals are bad for your body, no matter what—just like bad heart surgeries are bad for your body. By "bad root canal" I mean one that is not done properly, without using magnification to see the intricate details of the procedure and without proper cleansing of the tooth. That's like having a tooth with a cavity that's not completely cleaned. Eventually, it's going to break down and become harmful.

There are more sophisticated technologies in dentistry today than ever before. With 3-D analysis, we now have a better picture than ever about the condition of a tooth and whether a root canal is successful. And while I believe in doing what we can to save a tooth—as I think you probably know by now having read the previous chapters—sometimes, extraction is the only solution.

But removing a tooth for the sake of non-documented information about all root canals being bad opens up a whole new problem. An extraction is not a bacterial-free procedure. It still opens up the body to a different type of infection in the body. And resolving that can be very expensive compared to the cost of saving the tooth with a root canal—which may have been the best solution in the first place.

Deciding whether a tooth is salvageable comes down to a number of factors—how much tooth is remaining, where the infection is, how well that tooth can be cleaned up, and the technology that the person is using. And having the right person do those things makes all the difference in the world.

For Kevin,
Better Oral Health = Better Overall Health

The last time I visited with Kevin, he was planning his wedding. Getting his oral health back also helped him improve his overall health and let him move forward with a happier life.

Unfortunately, for many people, a fear of dentists is holding them back from having the kind of success that Kevin experienced. But it doesn't have to be that way. Let me tell you why in the next chapter.

SMILE ON!

What you can do now to improve your oral and overall health:

- Have a better diet with less carbonation, which is healthier for teeth and bones.

- Manage any increase of biofilm with regular dental cleanings and good home care.

- Be aware that many medications could increase dry mouth (causing decay), clenching, and tooth wear.

CHAPTER 10

THERE'S NO
REASON TO FEAR

Every day I see patients who remind me of my mom and her experiences, which reminds me about why I got into dentistry in the first place.

Millions of people are fearful about going to the dentist. Sadly, they delay vital dental care due to fears or negative past experiences at the dentist—their own or the experience of a friend or relative. When I started dental school, the statistic back then was that half of the population feared going to the dentist—and from what I've seen, that number hasn't changed much.

In fact, when their financial resources decrease, people sometimes become even more fearful about having dental work done. They're so worried about the costs that they won't even consider a dental visit for a cleaning. Many people delay essential care until the pain sends them to the emergency room. According to the American Dental Association: "Emergency rooms throughout the country have seen a dramatic increase in the number of patients seeking treatment for dental pain, from 1.1 million in 2000 to 2.1 million in 2010. The majority of these patients are suffering from dental decay that could easily have been prevented."[38]

The media doesn't help matters either. Several movies exaggerate a visit to the dentist. When I opened my practice in 1987, the movie *Little Shop of Horrors* came out with the memorable and cringeworthy storyline featuring a crazy dentist, played by actor Steve Martin. Plus, these days, there's so much misinformation online that anyone can find any story to back their fears.

If you're afraid of the dentist, you're not alone. But knowing some of these points can help you remove fear.

> **Not every dentist is the same.** There are many dentists who are empathetic and who listen carefully to patient concerns and address them with a more personal touch. At my practice, we take time to know each of our patients and we treat them in a blame-free manner. We try to understand why they are so stressed about going to the dentist. Our goal is to build a healthy relationship so that they can begin to trust us to do what's best for them.

> *"When I think of going to the dentist, so many emotions pop up for me. As a child, my earliest memory of my dentist was gold chains, too much cologne, and large fingers with rubber gloves that were sometimes not even changed between kids. Think Magnum P.I. meets Steve Martin's dentist character in* Little Shop of Horrors. *It was always a scary experience to get my teeth cleaned or a cavity filled because he truly had no compassion with kids being scared*

---

38   Laura Ungar, "ER Visits for Dental Problems Rising," *USA Today*, June 28, 2015, accessed March 20, 2019, www.usatoday.com/story/ newslocal/2015/06/24/er-visits-dental-problems-rising/29242113.

and was rough with how he handled you. I would have tears streaming down my face and he would just keep going with no desire to see how he could make me more comfortable.

"Fast forward to later years and I had to get my wisdom teeth removed. I remember the dentist standing over me trying to pull my teeth with all his might with drops of his sweat landing on my face. I had nothing but gas and Novocain, but he must have had the gas turned up to Mach 100 because I told him I was nauseous and, the next thing I know, I was throwing up halfway through the procedure. Needless to say, it was not a great experience. With all of this in my past, I went years without going to the dentist as an adult, even knowing I probably had issues that had to be addressed.

"Eventually, I had a few places that were bothering me badly enough that I knew I had gotten to the point that I had to give in. All the stars aligned in heaven and I found out about Dr. Flax. The first time I saw him, he was kind and patient, and he took the time to hear my story and do everything he could to make me comfortable. I would never go to anyone else because he has continually shown me that dentistry doesn't have to be painful or traumatizing. He has fixed everything from broken teeth, to root canals, to multiple crowns and fillings. My smile is now beautiful and I am so appreciative to have a dentist that I trust and consider a friend. I have been cured! (Just don't ever try to make me see anyone else.)"

—*Ashley Buero*

Pharmacological products can help. Some pharmacological products can aid in helping a patient with deep-seated fears.

Oftentimes, after many positive experiences, the patient will not have to depend on these medications for treatment.

Active participation in planning can eliminate surprises. When we build a healthy relationship with patients and they participate in their care, then there are no surprises. They know what's coming next, they know what to expect. And that can eliminate fear of the unknown.

Hence, collaboration is vital to your feeling in control. Knowing what cards you are dealing with will help you get some insight how to "play your hand" or knowing your options. There are benefits but also consequences and risks in whatever option you choose. Gaining the understanding helps you be aware of "what" your unique situation is, "why" it is helpful to you to care about it, and "how" to reach your goals as comfortably as possible.

No-drill dentistry equals no discomfort. In some cases, a hard-tissue laser can be used to remove decay (see chapter 6). The nature of these lasers is that they can alter the chemistry in a tooth so that, for a brief period of time, the tooth doesn't feel discomfort. Whether a laser is used for treatment depends on the case itself and factors such as tooth sensitivity or level of anxiety about going to the dentist. The laser can often eliminate the need for an anesthetic or for conscious sedation. If your fear of the dentist stems from the sound and vibrations from the dental drill, then drill-free dentistry may be right for you.

Sedation dentistry—a deep relaxation technique. Nitrous oxide (laughing gas) has been used to help people relax for many years. In addition, for some patients that are extremely anxious, there is a type of procedure known as **oral sedation**. The patient takes a dose of Triazolam (also known as a sleep aid called Halcion) that is a safe option for deep relaxation. It's a form of conscious sedation. But unlike general anesthesia, protective reflexes like breathing and coughing to clear the airway still function normally.

When the procedure is over, you may feel like you fell asleep, and you may have a little bit of amnesia. But you won't remember the dental procedure itself. As an added safety precaution, a trained professional monitors your vital signs, including pulse, heart rate, and oxygen levels, throughout the entire treatment.

With sedation dentistry, we can replace fillings or crowns, rejuvenate sore gums, fix a chipped tooth, and perform almost any dental procedure without fear or pain.

The nice thing about Triazolam medication is that, when it wears off, patients feel very refreshed. They don't feel hungover like they do from other sedative medications, such as Valium.

You may be a candidate for sedation dentistry if:

- you have had trouble getting numb during a dental treatment;

- you tend to gag when dental work is being done;

- you require extensive dental work. Sedation allows more treatment to be done in one sitting and can reduce the number of appointments needed;

- you experience anxiety or have had a bad experience with dentistry; and/or

- you put off regular care due to fear.

"Don't let past experiences or the media fuel any negative fire you have toward dentistry"

Another way to alleviate your fears is with **IV (intra-venous) Unconscious Sedation**. With specially trained professionals and advanced monitoring in a state board-approved facility, other medications will deepen your level of sedation so you sleep more profoundly. When your care is completed, you will be awake and still numb.

In both types of sedation, you must have someone drive you home after your care.

Bottom line: Don't put off your dental work any longer. That can make things worse. Without regular checkups, you run the risk of having dental infections that can lead to tooth loss and can even affect the health of the rest of your body.

Get to Know Your Dentist

Except where necessary, the goal with cosmetic dentistry is to be minimally invasive to create the smile you want. But, too often, patients put off having work done, and then the situation only worsens until the point that they have no other choice than to have more extensive—and more expensive—work done.

Instead, don't let past experiences or the media fuel any negative fire you have toward dentistry.

Look for a dentist with empathy for your situation. That's something easy for me to experience since I saw what my mom when through.

Becoming more aware and savvier about the options for your oral health care can help you find a dentist and practice that is well trained to serve you. Having the right dentist can relieve much of the anxiety you may be having about going in for treatment.

In the next chapter, we'll look for some of the secrets to finding your dream cosmetic dentist.

SMILE ON!

What can you do now to conquer your fears?

- Try hypnosis.

- Read reviews and testimonials from other people who have been able to conquer their fears with the right dentist.

- Seek a dental professional who has been trained and certified by DOCS Education (the Dental Organization for Conscious Sedation, www.docseducation. com).

- If you're looking for an improved smile, find a dentist that you can talk to, who listens to you, and that is experienced and credentialed with an organization such as the American Academy of Cosmetic Dentistry (AACD).

CHAPTER 11

THE SECRETS TO FINDING YOUR DREAM COSMETIC DENTIST

What exactly is a "dream cosmetic dentist"? It's an experienced and well-credentialed dentist that you can trust to deliver the smile you've longed for, a smile that you love and that will last a long time.

For many people, finding "Dr. Right" is a little like setting off on a journey. It can take months or even years to wade through all the online resources and dead-end referrals until they finally reach their destination—a dentist who they feel listens to them and offers creative solutions for their specific situation. In other words, their search for a dream cosmetic dentist is nothing short of a nightmare— and it can be an expensive one at that.

By the time I see patients, they're often so frustrated and frazzled that they're pretty much expecting the worst. So the first thing my team and I focus on is getting them comfortable with the whole idea of having dental work done. Then we take the time to gain a full understanding of what they're looking for in their smile, and we work collaboratively with them on the options available to help achieve those goals.

Rather than set off on a long, arduous journey in search of your dream dentist, start your search by taking into consideration these factors as ideal traits to look for your "Dr. Right."

Training and experience. Dentists typically complete the minimum number of continuing education (CE) hours required to maintain their license in the area in which they practice. On average, that's around twenty to thirty hours of CE each year. When looking for a cosmetic dentist, make sure that he or she completes at least the minimum hours of CE, and ideally exceeds those requirements. That demonstrates a passion for excellence and a desire to stay ahead of the curve when it comes to changes in this ever-evolving industry. On average, I complete 150 hours of CE each year, more than seven times the hours required by the State of Georgia.

Even better, find someone who is a leader in the field, someone that teaches others what they know *and* do. Someone who "walks the talk" and is considered a "KOL" (Key Opinion Leader) in dentistry. By **educator**, I mean someone who lectures regularly, authors articles, and/or tests innovative products. All are indicators of someone who is committed to continuous improvement, which will benefit you as a patient.

Credentialing. Look for dentists who are credentialed with one, if not all, of the major cosmetic dental organizations: with the American Academy of Cosmetic Dentistry (AACD), the American Academy of Esthetic Dentistry (AAED), and the American Society for Dental Aesthetics (ASDA). In Atlanta, I'm the only dentist who belongs to all three organizations, and I'm credentialed with the AACD and ASDA (the latter as Diplomate of the American Board of Aesthetic Dentistry), representing advanced training and experience, and the passing of an intensive examination by the credentialing board. *Though, at this time, there is no official specialty of cosmetic dentistry, certification of skills by objective and talented experienced peers is a good barometer for finding a great cosmetic dentist.*

Great communication skills. A practice whose team members listen first and are willing to collaborate with your care—can help improve the chances that you will have a great result. Often, you'll get even better results than you originally anticipated.

A team that has great communication skills will address your needs and desires, help you understand your treatment, and give you a reasonable idea of the time involved in getting your ultimate results so that you can best fit treatment into your schedule and budget.

Experience counts with a team that understands and advocates for you to help you get a realistic idea of what's achievable with your result. (Remember: Although cosmetic dentistry **"We help you** won't turn a senior into a teen again, it can take **understand your** years off your appearance.) That includes **options, and the pros** what's achievable when it comes to saving **and cons of each."** teeth. In my practice, we treat based on the evidence— the science of strengthening the functionality of your teeth and enhancing their appearance. We help you understand your options, and the pros and cons of each. So, where sometimes "conservative" treatment might mean sealing a tooth to protect it, that sealant or filling won't necessarily strengthen the tooth. Strengthening might involve another type of procedure altogether that will give you a better long-term result instead of patching up the tooth.

It's all about helping you understand your options so that you work with us to ensure you have the strongest, healthiest, and most functional smile possible.

Advanced technology. Look for a practice that's progressive, that's willing to use high technology to fully understand the details of your needs. In a field that's constantly evolving, and delivering better and better care, you want somebody who is not only constantly learning what the changes are and which are going to benefit their patients, but also bringing in the technologies to deliver the best care.

Through technologies such as digital scanning, 3-D printing, and photography, we gather data at the start of treatment, which helps us determine the optimal result for each patient. We also use advanced software to design your smile, which allows us to show your current and new smile on a chairside computer screen. Even better, this Digital Smile Design can help you test view a realistic mockup and preview how beautiful your smile could be. Lastly, with cone beam computed tomography (CBCT), we can get a 3-D image of a patient's bone structures, from the neck up. Those images can also help in treatment planning and outcomes—especially with implants. A future digital area that is growing is 3-D face scanning to fully visualize and plan a new smile while integrated with the items above. Keep an eye out for this new technique.

Utilizing laser technologies, we can gently sculpt gum tissue and to create a more-uniform, scalloped gumline. Lasers even allow us to offer anxiety-free treatments for issues such as tooth decay to help us restore teeth without anesthetic or dental drills.

And with tools such as the Kois Programmer and T-scan, we can balance out a bite to reduce tooth wear and fractures, allowing you to get long-term results.

Before-and-after patient pictures. I've had a number of patients show me photos from a dentist's website that are supposed to be before-and-after photos of their treatment cases. But I've seen the same photos in a number of places, including multiple websites and magazines.

When choosing the dentist for your treatment, make sure they have authentic photos of patients they have treated.

Smiles of the team. When vetting a dentist for your smile, look at the smiles of the members of the dentist's team. Often, the people that work in a cosmetic dental practice are essentially real-life examples of smile enhancements performed by the same dentist who could treat you.

Friendly, experienced team. Beyond the mechanics of the team members' smiles, also look for genuinely happy faces. A team that enjoys its work is more likely to make your experience one that you'll be happy you undertook.

No-fear atmosphere. In a no-fear office, you may actually feel a little spoiled. The dental team works to create a soothing atmosphere with friendly, smiling dental assistants and staff, and amenities such as warm neck pillows, comfy blankets for snuggling in during treatment, complimentary headsets for listening to music, and for waiting family members, refreshments and even a work area, if needed.

Proven lab tech. One of the keys to successful cosmetic dentistry is the relationship between the dentist and the lab technician who creates the restorations. Lab techs who are committed to creating natural-looking and long-lasting smiles takes extra pride in their work. And when they collaborate with the dentist, the result is the most ideal and realistic smile for the patient.

The lab should be well-equipped with the latest technologies, and understand which materials are ideal for your case. Ideally, they are also credentialed by the AACD and/or members of the AAED.

We've been working with the same cosmetic lab since 2000. It is based in California and is accredited with the AACD. Fortunately, with digital technologies that continue to evolve, we are able to synergistically plan cases to get better, longer-lasting outcomes for our patients. As our team concept continues to grow in a world of exponential changes, we've even learned from each other over the years.

Bottom line: You know you've found the right dentist when, from the very start of your visits, you feel that you are in a shared, positive relationship. That gives you peace of mind that all your concerns are being addressed, you have some control over your treatment, and as a result, you are destined to get the smile that you've dreamed of.

In short, if you've followed my advice, you'll know right away that you're going to love the way you look and how vibrantly healthy you feel for many years.

Once you have that amazing smile, it's time to keep it as long as you can.

SMILE ON!

What can you do now to begin your search for your
dream dentist?

- Take this book with you and follow the points in this
  chapter as you research for your dream dentist.

- Remember: Choosing a cosmetic dentist only by
  proximity to your home may not give you the results
  your desire.

- Go to DrHughFlax.com to learn more about all aspects
  of cosmetic dentistry.

ENJOYING YOUR SMILE FOR A LONG TIME— A HOW-TO GUIDE

Through the experiences I've shared with you about my mom and many of the patients at my practice, I hope you now see how important it is to have a beautiful smile, and how to make sure it's done right. Optimistically, you've found the stories I've shared with you to be a string of valuable pearls that help you make the informed right choices in your journey to have a smile that's the best it can possibly be. There's no need to fear when you have a dentist that's in your corner—someone who is experienced, cares about your comfort, and is working to ensure the best outcome for you.

A smile's not just about looking great in pictures, it's about feeling great in life. It's about walking into any room and people see a whole different way you carry yourself. It's about oozing happiness and having a greater level of confidence. That's not just on the outside, it comes from the inside. It's a combination of calm and energy that is indescribable. It's that "magic mojo" that everybody gets when they start feeling better about themselves.

Cosmetic dentistry is an investment in yourself—a healthier you.

A beautiful, believable smile is important. But having it last a long time for you and others to enjoy, is just as important. Form follows function when it comes to your smile: and you need to keep it healthy so it stays attractive for a long time.

Once you invest in rejuvenating your smile, you'll want to do everything to preserve it as long as possible. Some easy at-home tips to help you maintain a healthy smile include:

- twice daily brushing and thoroughly flossing at least once a day,

- using a low-abrasive toothpaste,

- minimizing carbonated drinks,

- maintaining a low-sugar intake, and

- regularly wearing your custom-designed bite guard to protect your teeth from friction and movement as well as relax your muscles and jaw joints.

Remember: Being proactive is one of the most important things you can do to have the smile you desire in order to minimize problems that could worsen over time. Oral health is just as important as overall health—when your mouth is healthy, you tend to live longer. You reduce your risks for heart disease, diabetes, obesity, and problems with pregnancies. To assist you, visiting your dentist as recommended is still a mainstay for your long-term wellness.

Another important thing to bear in mind: In order to advocate for your own health, you must also do that independently of what an insurance company says it will pay for your treatment. Letting the insurance company decide what kind of treatment you will receive is letting a non-dental professional decide what is right for you. It's very difficult to make the smart choices when you have an insurance company interfering with your health-care decisions.

During our voyage through this book, we've had a chance to explore the many tools we have available—from very conservative whitening, contouring, or bonding to long-lasting beautiful veneers to replacing missing teeth with implants. Just as important, we've covered "risk prevention" like bite balancing and wellness care to help your appearance improve and endure while keeping you very comfortable and relaxed.

The most important step you can take is to find a dentist who will always advocate for you—in every circumstance. The saddest thing in the world is for someone to feel like they've really done their homework in selecting a cosmetic dentist, but all they did was go to the internet and locate a practice nearby. Being knowledgeable will help you make the best decision on who can give you a beautiful smile that you will be happy to wear wherever you go.

On behalf of my mom and the many frustrated patients I've helped for almost forty years, I am grateful and applaud you for taking the time to read this book. It has truly been a labor of love.

As we finish our time here, I share this famous quote from Mahatma Gandhi:

"Be the change you wish to see in the world."

That is what I have tried to do throughout this book: help others gain the opportunity to enjoy excellent dental care and long-lasting, beautiful, believable smiles. We want you to confidently be able to say, "I love my smile!" and to feel better, look better, and enjoy a longer, healthier life.

You now possess the tools to control your destiny and make it happen. I hope I've given many of you a ray of hope to help you feel confident in your journey.

More importantly, I pray that you and many others will always find a *reason to smile* because of the promise I've sworn to keep.

GLOSSARY

Abfraction: Loss of tooth structure at the gumline causing concave or yellow areas where the root begins to show through.

Allograft: Sterilized cadaver bone used for grafting to create a foundation for implants. The safety of allografts is well documented, and protocols are strictly managed.

Autograft: The patient's own bone used for grafting for implants. The bone is dynamic and is typically taken from some area of the mouth.

Biofilm: The sludge of bacteria that permeates the body—including the mouth—that adheres to surfaces.

Bonding: Additive process that beautifies and strengthens tooth structure by impregnating natural microscopic porosities in the outer enamel and inner dentin with resin liquids called "bonding agents" allows them to become sticky enough to hold tooth-colored materials of varying strengths and colors.

Bruxing: Excessive grinding of the teeth that causes unnatural wear of the teeth.

Calculus: Hardened plaque on the teeth. Also known as **tartar**.

Cephalometric radiographs (x-rays): 2-D images of a patients face and teeth to help plan orthodontic treatment.

Cingulum: An anatomical feature on the back of the tooth. It keeps front teeth from flexing and breaking.

Cone Beam Computed Tomography (CBCT): A form of x-ray that delivers a 3-D image of the head and neck.

Contouring: A reductive procedure that reshapes natural tooth structure to make the teeth appear straighter.

Corticotomy: An accelerated and extremely predictable periodontal procedure that involves cutting the bone between teeth to move them orthodontically.

Crown: A dental restoration replacing the portion of the tooth above the gums. It can be made of varying materials, including porcelain or gold.

Dentin: The interior part of the tooth under the enamel or cementum.

Denture: A removable appliance that replaces multiple teeth and often covers the roof of the mouth, which can be bothersome to patients.

Embrasures: V-shaped valleys between adjacent teeth that help create the shape of the tooth (see picture in chapter 6).

Enamel: The visible white hard exterior of the tooth that protects the rest of the tooth during chewing. It is usually 2–3 mm when the tooth erupts and is vulnerable to breakdown from excessive friction from a heavy bite.

Equilibration: A gentle process of calibrating the bite so that the teeth uniformly contact when the jaws muscles are at rest.

Erosion: Loss of tooth structure due to chemicals that are often acidic.

Feldspathic: The classic porcelain made of glass used for cosmetic dentistry treatments, such as veneers or crowns. It is valued for its properties that make it closely resemble real teeth.

Fremitus: Palpable pathologic tooth vibration or micromovement caused by the teeth coming together or occluding.

Gingivitis: Gums that are swollen, puffy, tender, or bleed easily.

Grafting: A technique used to replace lost bone or gums.

Hybrid denture: An implant supported replacement that is connected to implants. Because it is "fixed," it is not bulky like a denture and feels more natural.

Implant: Artificial roots that are shaped like screws are placed in the jawbone. After they heal, they become a sturdy base for an artificial tooth or multiple teeth.

Laser: Technology that uses a beam of light to gently reshape gum and bone, as well as remove decay in a tooth. There are multiple strengths to serve each of these purposes. Special training is needed to use these safely and properly.

Lithium disilicate: A more modern type of porcelain used in cosmetic dentistry, for veneers, crowns, or conservative inlays/onlays. Valued for its strength and beauty and must be bonded.

Malocclusion: A bad bite where the teeth do not fit together well.

Nonaerobic bacteria: Bacteria that thrive without oxygen and tend to be deeper under the gums where the tissue is broken down.

Osseointegration: The process of an implant fusing to bone.

Overjet: An upper jaw that's too far forward.

Periodontitis: A severe form of gum disease that the supporting bone is lost.

Porosities: Refers to the porous surface of teeth.

Pressed ceramic: A modern type of fabricated material used in cosmetic dentistry. Valued for its beauty, strength, and accuracy.

Retainers: Appliances worn to keep teeth aligned after straightening with braces or aligners.

Temporomandibular joint (TMJ): The joints on either side of the face that connect the jawbone to the skull.

Tubules: Microscopic channels on teeth that lead to the nerves inside a tooth and allow them to feel heat and cold, and be affected by acidic substances.

Underbite: Characterized by lower teeth that are forward of upper teeth, often caused by excessive growth of the lower jaw.

Undercuts: The area of the tooth that dips in slightly and appears at the gumline.

Zirconia: A modern type of material used in cosmetic and restorative dentistry. Valued for its strength. Can look great esthetically, but often can be opaque, less translucent compared to natural teeth or tooth-colored tooth replacements like bonding or porcelains.

ABOUT THE AUTHOR

D r. Hugh Flax is internationally known for his leadership in cosmetic dentistry. A past president and accredited member of the American Academy of Cosmetic Dentistry (AACD), he has lectured and authored in Europe, Japan, Canada, and the United States on lasers, smile design, and advanced restorative techniques to enhance the skills of dental teams in making their care world class for their patients.

Dr. Flax is also a member of the editorial board of the Journal of Cosmetic Dentistry, a member of Catapult Education Speakers Group, and a certified Fellow with World Clinical Laser Institute, as well as the Academy of Laser Dentistry. He is founder of the Georgia Academy of Cosmetic Dentistry, and is a master with the International Congress of Oral Implantologists, an associate fellow of the American Academy of Implant Dentistry, a Diplomate of the American Board of Aesthetic Dentistry, a Kois Center graduate, a member of the American Academy of Esthetic Dentistry, and is in the CEREC Docs Continuum. In 2018, he joined the faculty of the AACD Residency Program in Cosmetic Dentistry.